CURANDERO

TRADITIONAL HEALERS OF MEXICO AND THE SOUTHWEST

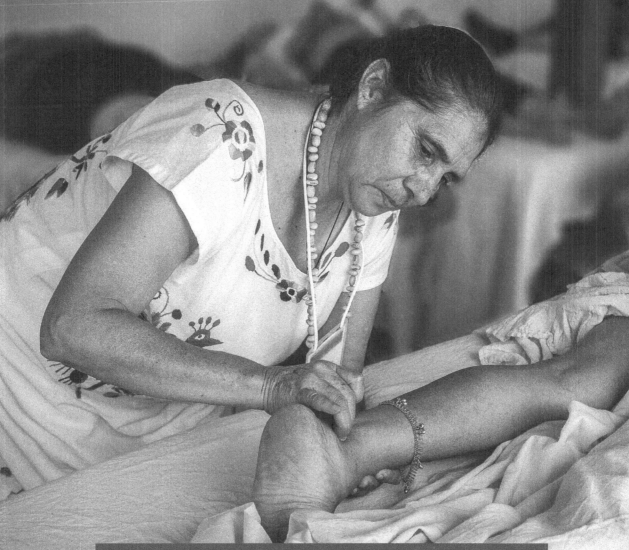

ELISEO "CHEO" TORRES ◉ IMANOL MIRANDA

Kendall Hunt
publishing company

Cover and interior images unless noted are courtesy of Imanol Miranda

Kendall Hunt
publishing company

www.kendallhunt.com
Send all inquiries to:
4050 Westmark Drive
Dubuque, IA 52004-1840

Published in the United States of America.

DEDICATION

We dedicate this book to many traditional healers from Mexico and the United States who have revived the tradition that has been part of the Hispanic/Latino culture for hundreds of years, *curanderismo*, the art of traditional medicine. Some of these knowledgeable, gentle, and kind healers have passed on to the spirit world, but their memories and contributions have touched the lives of hundreds of brothers and sisters in two bordering countries.

We also dedicate this book to the healers who present their knowledge and wisdom during the *curanderismo* course, the many students, participants, and the community members who have attended the class, and return to the classroom year after year to learn from the healers represented in this book.

We thank the many volunteers who organize a number of events related to the course, such as a traditional health fair and an herb walk at the Botanical Gardens of Albuquerque, and thank those behind the scenes who facilitate logistics, including moving furniture and providing food and transportation.

CONTENTS

INTRODUCTION

This book offers the contributions of a number of *curanderos(as)* (traditional healers) from two bordering countries, the United States and Mexico, through photographs by professional photographer Imanol Miranda, and narrated by Dr. Eliseo "Cheo" Torres, author and professor of the art of traditional medicine. For three years, Imanol attended the **Traditional Medicine without Borders: *curanderismo* in the Southwest and Mexico** two-week summer class taught by Dr. Torres at the University of New Mexico. This course attracts students, not only from New Mexico but also nationally and internationally, signifying a renewed interest in the field of traditional medicine, which has been somewhat lost and insufficiently researched, taught, or studied. Many of the students in the class recall how their grandmothers or relatives used medicinal plants and/or rituals for healing ailments. Unfortunately, the use of medicinal plants and the steps used in the rituals were not shared with the students because this tradition was not usually written, but rather passed down by word of mouth (often from mother to daughter) and distorted through time. The course, as well as the production of videos featuring healers participating in the class, allowed Dr. Torres to develop a semester-long online course on a number of rituals, healing therapies, demonstrations, and correct information regarding the use of medicinal plants. The photographs taken by Imanol and enjoyed by you are of many of the healers who taught in the summer class and/or were videotaped for the online class.

Imanol was able to capture the healers teaching class, performing a ritual, participating in a ceremony, or offering a healing session during a traditional health fair that was part of the summer *curanderismo* course.

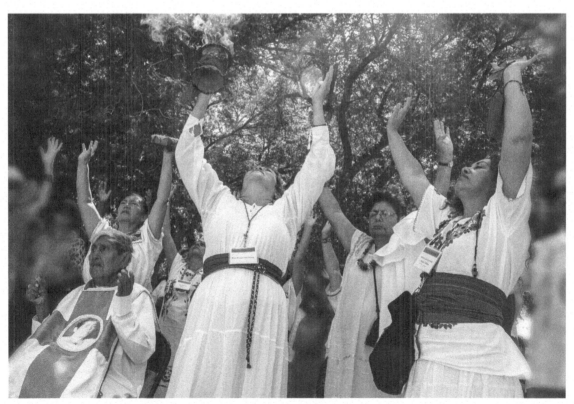

Honoring the four directions is part of an opening ceremony prior to traditional events or before entering a *temazcal* sweat lodge. In this case, healers such as Chenchito and Rita are joined by other *curanderos(as)* and students for a morning blessing before participating in a public health fair.

Many of the healers from Mexico such as Rita, Laurencio, Tana, Juan Carlos, Doris, and Lety mentored younger American professionals wanting to incorporate some of the rituals and traditional therapies into their practices. Because of the influence of the Mexican *curanderos(as)*, American healers such as Toñita and Laura have been practicing traditional medicine for years and have constructed Mexican sweat lodges called *temazcales*. Both healers teach and mentor groups of interns from Albuquerque and other parts of the country and meet with them on a regular basis to learn the traditional ways of healing and the powerful use of the sweat lodge to heal the body, mind, and spirit.

This publication begins with an overview of *curanderismo* including the definition, a brief history, influences, types of *curanderos*, and levels of healing. It continues with an explanation of how it has been revived at the national level by individuals such as Dr. Andrew Weil from the United States and Arturo Ornelas from Mexico.

We have divided this publication into chapters corresponding to four groups of healers. We call the first group ***Curanderos(as)* of Yesterday: The Three Great Ones**, after those who contributed to *curanderismo* in a different era, the late 1800s and early 1900s.

The second group is labeled as ***Curanderos(as)* of Recent Times: Impacting the United States and Mexico.** These four healers had an influence in Mexico and in the United States and have all died within the past few years. The third group is the largest number of healers in this book. Most are from Mexico and the United States with the exception of one from Puerto Rico. You will enjoy their biographies, photographs, and captions of what we call ***Curanderos(as)* of Nowadays: Creating a New Traditional Healing Model.** Most of the Mexican *curanderos(as)* devote much of their time to their healings and have established clinics, while the American healers have incorporated traditional healing modalities into their professions.

The fourth group is classified as ***Curanderos(as)* of Tomorrow** and consists of a small group of young professionals who are devoted to helping their communities by discovering and reclaiming their culture in traditional healing. Like the third group of healers, these professionals have incorporated traditional therapies into their practice and are determined to create a new paradigm of health services in merging modern with traditional healing.

Imanol Miranda

At the age of thirteen, Imanol moved with his parents and brothers to South Texas from Mexico City. Before that, they lived in the cities of Acapulco and Reynosa, Mexico. His parents introduced him to painting and photography from an early age. Following the tradition of his parents, Imanol chose to obtain a Bachelor of Fine Arts degree with emphasis on photography and graphic design. He spent many hours studying the paintings of masters such as Raphael, Michelangelo, Titian, Rembrandt, Peter Paul Rubens, and Nicolas Poussin. Those paintings inspired Imanol to produce compelling photographs that explore the complexities of the human experience.

His passion for photography led him to meet Dr. Eliseo "Cheo" Torres in 2014. Imanol accepted Dr. Torres' invitation to photograph the *Traditional Medicine without Borders: Curanderismo in the Southwest and Mexico* course at the University of New Mexico. Imanol agreed because he wanted to reconnect with his Mexican roots and explore the stories of Mexican American people in the United States. His previous photographs on Mexican American culture have been displayed at prominent cultural venues in South Texas as well as at the Emma S. Barrientos Mexican American Cultural Center in Austin.

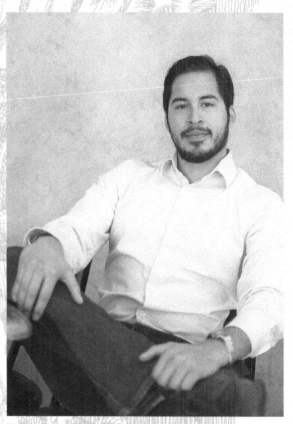

Photographer, Imanol Miranda, has a passion for using photographs to tell the cultural stories of the Latino/Hispanic culture such as the art of traditional medicine, *curanderismo*. Photo credit: Melissa Barzaga.

Eliseo "Cheo" Torres

Since he was a boy growing up near the border of Texas and Mexico, Eliseo Torres, known to everyone as "Cheo," has been fascinated by the folk traditions and folkways of Mexico and of his Mexican American roots. Both of his parents were versed in aspects of herbal lore and healing, and as he matured he learned from them a love and respect for the history and knowledge of the ancient art of Mexican folk healing. Cheo regularly lectures and gives presentations on the history and lore of *curanderismo* to audiences ranging from scholars and students of Latin American culture to people hoping to become knowledgeable about alternative and traditional medicine. He has published two books on his life and research: **Curandero: A Life in Mexican Folk Healing** and **Healing with Herbs and Rituals: A Mexican Tradition.** He teaches at the University of New Mexico (UNM) a two-week course and an online class on the topic of *curanderismo*.

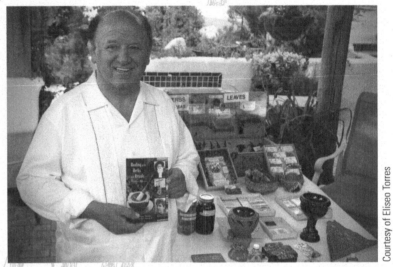

Courtesy of Eliseo Torres

Author, Dr. Eliseo "Cheo" Torres, has been teaching a class on the traditional medicine of Mexico and the Southwest for almost 20 years.

An Overview of *Curanderismo*

CHAPTER 1

What Is *Curanderismo?*

In order to appreciate the action photographs of a number of *curanderos(as)* from Mexico and throughout the United States in this publication, it is important to understand the traditional healing culture that has played a role in the health of Hispanics/Latinos in the two bordering countries.

Curanderismo is the art of Mexican folk healing and comes from the Spanish word "*curar*" meaning "to heal." It is a holistic approach to healing by treating and assessing an individual's body, mind, and spirit (some *curanderos(as)* and healers often refer to spirit as "energy"). To become a *curandero(a)*, in earlier years, a person could apprentice under an existing healer and/or have some kind of healing gift, or "*don*" as it is referred to in Spanish. Currently, there are schools such as *El Centro de Desarrollo Humano Hacia la Comunidad*/The Center for Community Human Development in Cuernavaca, Mexico, which prepare students interested in this field of study and offer training to practicing *curanderos(as)* in various healing therapies. Recently, in the United States, *curanderismo* therapies have transformed and are incorporated into other professions such as nursing, massage, ministry, and even mainstream medicine. This phenomenon is occurring in states such as New Mexico and Minnesota, which you will be able to appreciate through the photographs of the practitioners featured in this book. Please note that the word "*curandero*" is used when referring to a male healer, while a "*curandera*" is used for a female. Following Spanish grammar, when this book refers to a group of *curanderos,* we are including both male and female healers in that grouping.

Brief History of *Curanderismo*

In order to understand where *curanderismo* stands in a modern setting, we need to understand its origin. Mexico is a country of rich cultural heritages. Numerous indigenous populations that lived in the region for thousands of years learned about and utilized the plants, animals, and environment around them to treat and prevent physical ailments. Aztec herbology was vast and comprehensive, hundreds of years before the Spaniards arrived in Mexico. It is important to understand Spain's history as well. Spain is a region that had settlements dating back into prehistory and long before the eventual invasion by the Roman Empire. Following the Muslim and Moorish conquest of Spain in 718 CE to about 1031 CE, Muslim, Jewish, and Christian populations grew and lived together in harmony. The regions exchanged cultural practices, loaned words from various languages, and shared healing modalities.

By the time Spaniards arrived in Mexico in 1519, the culturally complex worlds of the Spanish and the indigenous peoples collided. Unfortunately, this destroyed an opportunity for another great multicultural renaissance. As a result, by 1521, Tenochtitlan, the capital city of the Aztec empire, was destroyed, and with it, apparently, the Aztec knowledge of over 3,000 medicinal plants.

In 1552, 31 years after the conquest of Mexico, Martin de la Cruz, an Aztec doctor, wrote the first medical journal in the New World since the conquest, a book entitled **Codex Badiano** (named after his scribe, Juan Badiano). The Codex Badiano listed 251 herbs and medicinal plants at the School of Santa Cruz de Tlatelolco. In 1554, Cervantes de Salazar described Montezuma II's gardens while physicians experimented with hundreds of medicinal herbs.

The Codex Badiano was printed on amaté paper made from the amaté tree, and was translated from the Aztec language of Nahuatl to Latin. It features detailed color illustrations of plants, as well as their Nahuatl names. Unfortunately, the Codex Badiano was lost to Mexico for four centuries. In 1990, it was returned to Mexico when Pope John Paul II visited there, and it now resides at Mexico City's National Institute of Anthropology and History. There is still a strong usage of medicinal plants throughout Mexico, with some coming from the old world and others already here in the new world.

Some of the main lineages of *curanderismo* are as follows:

1. **Native American and Spanish** roots date back to the arrival of the Spanish explorers and missionaries when their knowledge of traditional Moorish medicine was blended with that of the natives of the New World.

2. **Judeo-Christian** roots came with the Spaniards, including the Christian belief that healing is a gift of God and the parts of the healing treatment that combine prayer with ritual.

3. **Greek Humoral Medicine** is based on the theory of the equilibrium of hot and cold, and the treatment is based on bringing a balance of temperature to the body. It is similar to the yin and yang Chinese theory that treats hot illnesses with cold remedies and vice versa.

4. **Arabic and Islamic** beliefs recognize psychic energy, which a person can use to send mental vibrations to another person thereby causing illness. The Spaniards borrowed this belief from the Moorish culture that dominated Spain for 800 years and brought it to the new world. An example of this influence is *mal de ojo* (evil eye), the negative vibrations that come from a jealous gaze. It is treated by performing a *limpia*.

5. **African** Caribbean *Santeria Orichas (African Spirits)* are blended with Catholic saints. *Limpias* are also a part of the healing repertoire.

6. **Spiritualism and Psychic** trances and communication with spirits are part of the *Fidencista* movement of the followers of Niño Fidencio, the famous *curandero* who died in 1938. This may have been influenced by French educator and author, Allan Kardec. In the mid-1800s, he studied psychic phenomena and wrote, "The Spirit Book." Chenchito, featured in this publication, channels the spirit of Niño Fidencio during some of his healings.

7. **Scientific** influence is evident with many of the healers in this publication who also teach in a holistic medicine school in Cuernavaca. Such healers know germ theory, psychology, and biomedicine, and collaborate with physicians and nurses. In this book, there are a number of photographs of American allied health professionals from around the country who are incorporating medicinal plants and rituals into their practices.

Some Types of *Curanderos*

1. *Sobador(a)* —a folk masseur(se) who specializes in *Sobadita* which is used on a sprain. A *masaje* is a total full-body massage and many times is the first step in the healing process. A *sobador(a)* may listen to the patient's problems during the massage in order to determine whether the illness is physical, mental, or both. A benefit of a massage is the reduction of cortisol, the body's stress hormone, and the release of endorphins, the body's natural painkiller.

2. *Temazcalero(a)*—a guide to a traditional *temazcal* or sweat lodge. At times, a *curandero(a)* may specialize as a *temazcalero(a)*. These sweat lodges were dying out, but are now returning to Mexico and the United States. The following chapters include images of sweat lodges and of the *curanderos(as)* who are preserving the tradition.

3. *Huesero(a)*—a bonesetter, usually without formal training, who practices in a way similar to that of a *sobador(a)* or chiropractor, but focuses on the bones and joints of a person, and getting them into the correct alignment. In the modern world, there are very few *hueseros*. *Huesero* Agustin Pérez is featured in this publication.

4. *Partera*—a *curandera* that specializes in midwifery. There is a photograph in this publication of Dr. Felina Ortiz, who is a *partera* as well as university faculty.

5. *Yerbero(a)* —a *curandero(a)* who uses herbs and is considered a master herbalist. Many of the healers in this publication are also *yerberos(as)*, specifically Doris Ortiz and Katherine White.

6. *Curandero(a) Total*—a healer who is gifted at all of the specialities within *curanderismo*. Examples in this publication are Rita Navarrete and Toñita Gonzales.

7. *Materia/cajita*—the term used by the followers of the *Fidencista* movement who incorporate many of the therapies in addition to channeling spirits such as that of the famous healer *Niño Fidencio*. Chenchito, whom you will learn about, is a *materia/cajita*.

Another well-known practice in *curanderismo* is the *limpia* or spiritual or energetic cleansing ritual. Almost all *curanderos* incorporate the *limpia* into their practice, but some specialize in it. In this publication, you will see photographs of a number of healers performing *limpias* using different elements such as *copal* incense, plants, and feathers.

Levels of the Self in *Curanderismo*

Based on my studies in the field and the teachings of many traditional healers I have met, *curanderos*, folk healers, shamans, and medicine men primarily work on three different levels: the material, the spiritual, and the mental. The material level involves a person's physical body and the ailments, pains, and diseases that affect it physically (i.e., stomach ache, arthritis, sciatica). The spiritual (also referred to as energetic) level involves a person's soul or where are they spiritually. Ailments in this area range from a person feeling lost, feeling like they need spiritual protection from bad energy, or grieving the death of a loved one. *Limpias* are the most common rituals that address the spiritual level. The mental level involves anything psychological that is affecting a person in a negative way such as the inability to focus, low self-esteem, insomnia, and/or depression. This level is the most difficult one to address, and the healer may channel mental vibrations to the patient to help in the healing process. Elena Avila, Felipa Sánchez, and Chenchito are three healers who were effective in the mental level of healing.

In *curanderismo*, many healers use religious and supernatural levels, such as prayers, in conjunction with healing rituals. Chenchito and Felipa Sánchez use prayer in all of their healings. Some healers prefer to use the term energy instead of spirit or soul, and natural descriptions such as Mother Earth, Father Sky, and the Creator, in lieu of God.

Curanderos observe, study, and work with one, two, or any combination of the material, spiritual, and mental levels. On the physical level, the *curandero* will use plants, candles, oils, incense, tinctures (alcohol-based remedies that use fresh or dried herbs or plants), microdosages, called *microdosis* in Spanish (water-based remedies made from tinctures), and amulets which vary from culture to culture and are usually small objects that offer protection for an individual or home, but can also be used for good health, good luck, or may have very specific purposes.

On the spiritual level, a *curandero* will serve as a "medium" to mediate between the patient and parts of his/her soul or soul concept. The belief is that a patient may have lost their soul, or part of their spirit. The late *curandera*, Elena Avila, referred to the cure for this as a soul retrieval, a form of shamanic work in which she tried to retrieve the soul of the person. Afterwards, the person would feel better, renewed, and whole again. The *limpia* and a *plactica* (a counseling session) can be included at this level. On the mental level, the *curandero(a)* will channel mental vibrations to the patient. This can be observed in rituals such as *mal de ojo*, which will be discussed shortly.

Popular Plants Used at Material Level

The following is a list of popular plants used by *curanderos*. Due to the similarities in names and plant families across the world, it is always best to double-check which herbs you are using and use caution when referring to the Spanish or English common names, keeping in mind that the names change according to regions of the country. However, the Latin scientific botanical names never change, such as those included in this section.

1. **Arnica** has the same name in English and Spanish. The botanical or Latin name is *Arnica Montana,* and it can be used for many ailments including, but not limited to, insect bites, sprains, and wounds.

2. *Chaya*, *Cnidoscolus chayamansa,* sometimes referred to as the spinach tree, is used as a nutritional supplement as it is richer in vitamins, calcium, and iron than spinach and alfalfa. It is a diuretic, has anti-diabetic properties, and is used to help control type II diabetes.

3. **Damiana**, *turnera diffusa,* is used for anxiety, asthma, colic, mild indigestion, and a popular aphrodisiac sometimes referred to as the "natural viagra."

4. *Manzanilla* (Spanish), or **chamomile** (English), is known by the scientific name *Matricaria Recutita* and has a wide range of uses, including anti-inflammatory properties, treating anxiety, colic, fever, headaches, insomnia, nausea, as a sedative, and an eyewash.

5. *Romero*/**rosemary**, *Rosmarinus officinalis,* is used for treating symptoms of Alzheimer's and can be used as a memory booster, circulation enhancer, menstruation enhancer, and postpartum bath. It is a very drought-tolerant plant and grows nicely in New Mexico, especially in the Albuquerque area.

6. **Tepezcohuite**, *Mimosa tenuiflora,* has no English translation. It is found in Brazil, but also Oaxaca and Chiapas, Mexico. It is a Central and South American tree that is used for acne, burns, scars, wound healing, and wrinkles. It is very popular in Mexico and is almost always used topically.

7. *Tila*/**linden tree,** *Tilia cordata,* is used to treat depression, headaches, insomnia, and restlessness, and is used as a mild sedative.

8. *Uña de gato*/**cat's claw,** *Uncaria tomentosa,* is the Peruvian type from the Amazon Rainforest and should not be confused with the American cat's claw or some Mexican varieties that can be toxic. This Peruvian plant is anti-inflammatory, a kidney cleanser, is used for viral infections and wound healing, and is an immunosuppressant. Once a person's immune system strengthens, their health improves.

9. *Yerba buena*/**spearmint**, *Mentha spicata,* is one of the most common and popular herbs used by *curanderos(as)*. It is used to treat colds, for digestive aid, to treat headaches, indigestion, and for nausea.

Other Elements of the Material Level

Another facet of the material level is the use of candles. Different-colored candles signify different needs, intentions, or desired effects. Sometimes, the way that the flames will flicker or the way the wax melts can be read and interpreted by certain *curanderos* to identify and treat certain ailments or illnesses. Generally, blue is used for serenity, pink for goodwill, white for purity, red to help treat illness and for love, while green and black candles attack negative forces.

Type of Spiritual and Mental Levels

Although they are two separate levels, the spiritual and mental will be described as one in this section since they are difficult to separate. On the spiritual and mental levels, a *curandero(a)* works with a patient with various conditions, such as *mal de ojo*/the evil eye, *susto*/fright, sometimes called magical fright, *caida de mollera*/fallen fontanel, which is the soft part of a baby's head, *empacho*/intestinal blockage, *bilis* and *muina.* *Bilis* is suppressed anger causing excessive bile in the system. *Muina i*s outward rage causing an inability to talk, at times.

Common Conditions Treated by *Curanderos*

Mal Ojo—It is referred to as the evil eye and is commonly defined as one person glaring or staring at another person, usually a baby. It can cover other forms of excessive attention. Commonly, *mal de ojo* is caused by an excessive admiration. For example, an attractive person or an infant whose immune system is weak can be the recipient of *mal de ojo* even though the intention is not negative. All of the energy fixated on that one person can cause disharmony. Treatment for *mal de ojo* is one of the most common reasons people seek out a traditional healer.

Susto—Some refer to it as magical fright, and it is caused by a traumatic experience. Some extreme fright could be related to post-traumatic stress disorder (PTSD). Car accidents can be a source of *susto* for both of those involved and for witnesses. Some professions such as soldiers, clergy, police officers, and firefighters are more susceptible to experience *susto*.

Caida de mollera—Translated as fallen fontanelle, it can be caused when a baby is tossed in the air or if the baby falls from the crib. The fontanelle is the soft spot on top of the baby's head that can cave in. The idea is to raise it again.

Empacho —This is a bolus of food lodged in a digestive tract that causes intestinal blockage and constipation as a result of swallowing chewing gum or foods that are raw or not fully cooked. This usually happens to babies who crawl and eat contaminated items from the floor.

Revival of *Curanderismo*

Today, *curanderismo* has influenced the revival of alternative, complementary, holistic, or integrated medicine and includes millions of dollars in consumer spending. This money is spent on traditional therapies and herbal preparations used by healers. Dr. Andrew Weil, sometimes called the "guru of alternative medicine," promotes the idea that "If it can't hurt you, it could help you." Weil suggests dietary approaches to health such as eating less fat, animal products, managing stress, eliminating or reducing intake of alcohol, cigarettes, and coffee, and beginning various forms of exercise, massage, and hypnosis therapy. He also recommends the use of herbs such as garlic, ginger, and cooking with olive oil. He suggests using medicinal herbs and keeping lots of fresh flowers around. Weil believes that having fresh flowers around can be very therapeutic. His philosophy and recommendations mirror, in many ways, what *curanderos(as)* have always practiced and preached. They promote the dietary approaches that Dr. Weil recommends as is evident in many of their therapies. Many of the *curanderos(as)* eat and recommend a healthy lifestyle of balanced meals and the avoidance of alcohol and cigarettes. Most of them perform traditional massage therapy called *sobadas* and prescribe plant remedies. Most of them keep fresh flowers in their homes and clinics and even prescribe them as part of their healings. In many ways, they have been ahead of Dr. Weil's philosophy of healing.

In addition to the work that Dr. Andrew Weil has done in reviving integrated medicine, another champion in Mexico has been promoting traditional holistic medicine for more than 30 years. Dr. Arturo Ornelas received his doctorate at the University of Geneva, Switzerland, and did field health work with the Latin American World Health Organization before returning to Mexico to establish the Center for Community Human Development/*Centro de Desarrollo Humano Hacia la Comunidad*, an institute and school that offers holistic traditional medicinal instruction

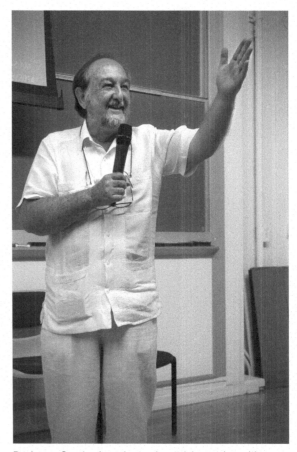

Dr. Arturo Ornelas is a pioneer in studying and teaching traditional medicine. He founded a unique school recognized by the Mexican government, which is located in the city of Cuernavaca, Morelos, Mexico. The school also has branches in Mexico City, Mérida, and other cities in Mexico.

to hundreds of healers from Mexico and throughout the world. His institute has revived many of the lost traditional therapies and has improved the quality of life for many by offering certificates and diplomas in traditional and integrated medicine.

The instructors of his school, who are also healers, have established a number of health clinics throughout Mexico and teach short courses on traditional medicine in their communities. The same teachers participate in the University of New Mexico summer *curanderismo* course and are shown in photographs throughout this publication.

A number of U.S. professionals have been trained by the Mexican instructors/healers in various traditional therapies and now have incorporated these methods into their healing practices. This group is now reviving methods that have been lost, and you will enjoy their photographs in this book.

In the previous image, Dr. Ornelas addresses and welcomes the students of the *curanderismo* class at the University of New Mexico. He has been partnering with Dr. Torres for many years to offer the class. In addition, both have produced an online course that is taken worldwide. Some of the students in these courses choose to further their education by studying at Dr. Ornelas' institute.

Three great *curanderos*, whom I referred to as, "Three Great Ones"/*Los Tres Grandes,*" have also influenced modern *curanderismo*. The three include Don Pedrito Jaramillo (1829–1907), Teresita (1873–1906), and Niño Fidencio (1898–1938).

Don Pedrito Jaramillo was also called the "Healer of Los Olmos" (Los Olmos is a ranch outside of Falfurrias, Texas) and was one of the most powerful men in the Southwest during his lifetime. Jaramillo adopted a son, Severiano Barrera, rumored to have been given to Jaramillo as a token of appreciation from a couple that he healed. Barrera would answer a lot of Don Pedrito's correspondence and was investigated by the U.S. Post Office because there were more stamps going out of Los Olmos than the U.S. Post Office had brought in. They discovered that Jaramillo had a barrel full of stamps and self-addressed envelopes from people writing him, indicating his popularity as a healer. Why were his prescriptions simple remedies such as water, baths, and mud? It could have been because people were poor back then and could not afford to purchase medications or Don Pedrito was testing their faith with these plain remedies.

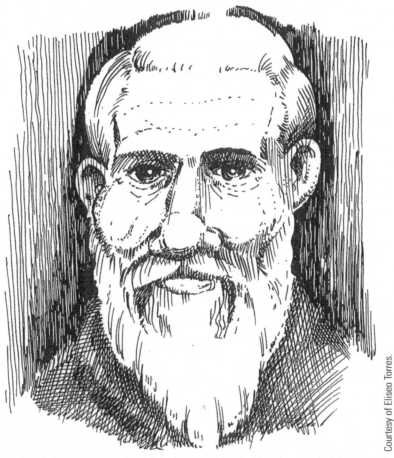

Courtesy of Eliseo Torres.

Don Pedrito Jaramillo was known as the healer of Los Olmos, a community located near Falfurrias, Texas. He died in 1907.

Teresita Urrea died at the age of 33 and was thought of as a folk saint of her region. This is why she was called Santa Teresita, but was not a canonized saint recognized by the Catholic Church. She was the illegitimate daughter of a poor native peasant and wealthy aristocratic rancher. She apprenticed under an older *curandera* by the name of Huila and utilized powers of hypnosis and prophecy. When Teresita was nineteen, she was exiled from Mexico by President Porfirio Diaz who referred to her as a "dangerous agitator." Diaz sent 500 armed men to enforce the exile. Teresita fled to Nogales, Arizona, and then moved to El Paso, Texas, where she healed 200 patients a day. Rebels attacking Mexico from New Mexico called themselves *Teresistas* in her honor and wore pictures of her pinned to their shirts. She is buried in Clifton, Arizona.

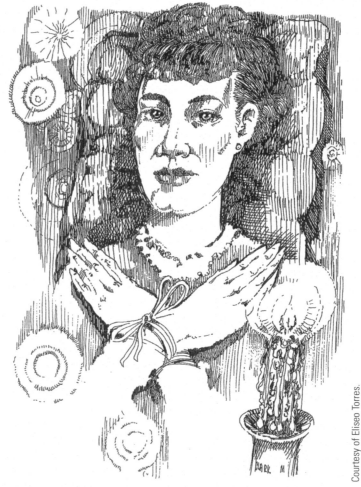

Courtesy of Eliseo Torres.

Teresita went into a coma after an attempted rape and was thought to be dead. She was dressed for burial with her hands bound across her breasts and suddenly woke-up puzzled by her funeral. She died in 1906.

Niño Fidencio whose full name was Jose Fidencio de Jesus Constantino Sintora was nicknamed *"Niño"* as a term of endearment for being innocent and childlike. He was always happy and laughing.

It is said that Fidencio cured President Plutarco Elias Calles and his daughter of a terrible illness and became famous after the story was reported in the newspapers. He is linked to Jesus Christ since he had disciples, performed cures, wore a tunic, and walked barefoot. El Niño prescribed laughter with the approach that people are not as sick as they think they are and would often say, "here let's have a laugh and you'll feel better." He is honored with two celebrations in the small community of Espinazo in Northeast Mexico. Chenchito is a Fidencista, a follower of Niño Fidencio, channels his spirit, and has a home in Espinazo, where El Niño lived and is buried. Chenchito is featured in this book.

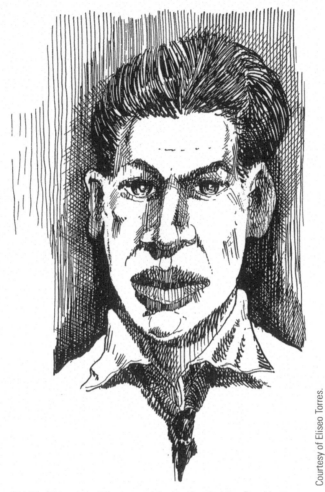

Courtesy of Eliseo Torres.

El Niño Fidencio, of Espinazo, Mexico, healed the President, Plutarco Elias Calles. He died in 1938.

There are some commonalities between *Los Tres Grandes*: All three were considered somewhat different and odd; they never charged a fee, but accepted donations; and they were all noble, sincere, and humble. They were charismatic leaders with great followings and were considered folk saints while still alive (saints of the people and not recognized by the church). According to folk belief, El Niño and Teresita were both 33 (in reality El Niño was not 33, but some want to believe he was the same age as Jesus Christ) when they died and all had the power of prophecy. Some say that Don Pedrito was the Oral Roberts of his time since he healed through faith; Teresita was the Jean Dixon of her time since she healed through hypnosis and prophecy; and El Niño was the Norman Cousins of his time since he healed people through laughter. All three requested their coffins to be opened three days after their deaths, but this was never done.

Curanderos(as) of Recent Times: Impacting the United States and Mexico

Some well-known *curanderos(as)* who have made an impact in both the United States and Mexico are as follows: Jewel Babb from Valentine, West Texas, Elena Avila from Albuquerque, New Mexico, Alberto Salinas, Jr. from Edinburg, Texas, and Felipa Sánchez from Mexico, with a part-time clinic in Albuquerque. All of these well-known and generous healers have passed on, but left an impressive legacy of their contributions in touching the lives of many people in at least two countries. Jewel is considered the "Goat Woman of West Texas." She discovered healing power at the age of 56, and her faith and prayers to God were part of her healings. She did traditional massage therapy, prescribed medicinal herbs, and did not charge for her services. Her clients were from both the United States and Mexico since she lived on the border of both countries. I was so impressed with Jewel that I went to visit her in Valentine, Texas, but because of her illness she could not see me. Soon after my visit, she passed away.

Elena Avila was a well-known *curandera* who specialized in *platicas*/counseling talks, and various types of spiritual cleansing rituals using eggs, feathers, and plants. She was a registered nurse who worked in a psychiatric hospital and later became a *curandera*. Elena considered herself an heir to the ancient Aztec healing traditions and was particularly powerful and effective in her treatment of women's traumas. She worked with a number of *curanderas(os)* in Mexico and collaborated with the Center for Community Human Development in Cuernavaca. She touched the lives of many patients and students that she mentored throughout the United States before passing away in her sleep in 2011. We often visited to share some good conversations, and she is a dear friend, who is missed.

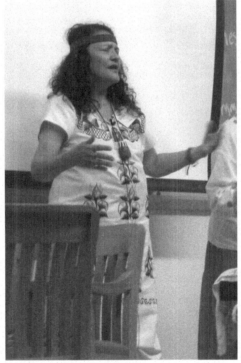

Courtesy of Dorene DiNaro.

Elena Avila at the University of New Mexico.

I never met Alberto Salinas, Jr., but communicated with him by phone and mail. He was a well-known *materia,* a title given to a *curandero(a)* who practices the Fidencista tradition. This is the same title that my teacher and mentor, Chenchito, uses. Alberto was well known in Espinazo, Mexico, where he spent time attending the annual healing festivals honoring Niño Fidencio. He served clients from both the United States and Mexico in his clinic located on the border town of Edinburg, Texas. He coauthored the book "*Curandero* Conversations" with my friend and colleague Dr. Antonio Zavaleta. In his second book, "El Niño Fidencio and the Fidencistas: Folk Religion in the U.S.-Mexican Borderland," Dr. Zavaleta recognizes him with the following words: "Alberto died in 2013, a man of vast experience and ability, for he was a well read and highly informed man of native intelligence. He understood my research perfectly and often anticipated my questioning offering more than I expected and new lines of investigation. Unlike most other *materias* of El Niño Fidencio, Alberto had an acute understanding of the role that *curanderos* play in border society and therefore he wanted to be recognized for his contribution and was often rewarded with interviews statewide. Toward the end of his life, I assisted him in publishing a book chronicling his life as a border healer." Alberto Salinas Jr.'s legacy will continue because of his writings and support by Dr. Antonio Zavaleta.

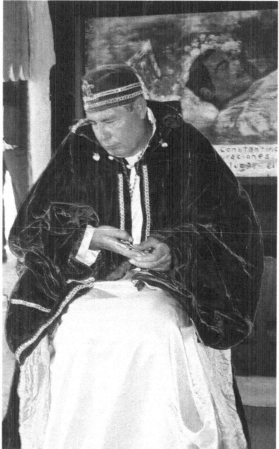

Courtesy of Alberto Salinas Jr.

Alberto Salinas Jr.

Felipa Maria Magdalena Sánchez was loved by many clients and friends from the United States and Mexico. She was a tribal leader in her Mazahua native community of San Felipe del Progreso and a teacher of *curanderismo* at the holistic medicine school in Cuernavaca. She traveled to California and New Mexico to serve a number of clients and to deliver workshops to students of traditional medicine. A well-known herbalist and healer in Albuquerque, Maclovia Sánchez de Zamora, established a clinic in her herb store, Ruppe Drugs, for a number of years where Felipa served the community by doing body adjustments, spiritual cleansings, and prescribing herbal medications. Felipa was a devoted *curandera* and faith healer, and was considered a clairvoyant because of her ability to see beyond the physical. She passed away on a return trip from Albuquerque to her Mexican community of San Felipe del Progreso.

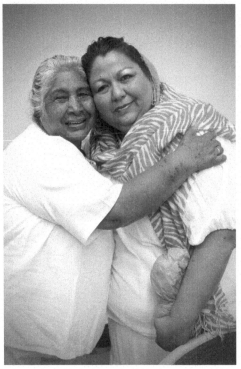

Felipa Sánchez (left) and Toñita Gonzales (right)
at the University of New Mexico.

Even though these four healers have passed on to the spirit world, they had some commonalities, just like the healers of yesteryear. All were humble, gentle, and sincere, they gave credit for their healings to the Creator, they were teachers and mentors to others, and all were charismatic leaders. Publications were written about all three beginning with Elena Avila's book, **Woman Who Glows in the Dark**; Alberto Salinas Jr. was the writer of **The Border Healer: My Life as a *Curandero*** and the coauthor of ***Curandero* Conversations**; and in addition, **Border Healing Woman** is the story of Jewel Babb.

Curanderos(as) of Nowadays: Creating a New Traditional Healing Model

We have learned of ***Curanderos(as) of Yesteryear,*** whom I refer to as "The Three Great Ones/*Los Tres Grandes*" because of their contributions to healing in the late 1800s and early 1900s. In some ways, they were ahead of their times with therapies such as healing with water, which is now called hydrotherapy and is used by many therapists. They also healed with laughter, which is called Laugh Therapy, is practiced in many hospitals, and taught by healers like Rita Navarrete. They all prescribed medicinal herbal plants which are the basis for many modern medications and are used by all the healers featured in this publication. All three *curanderos(as)* were popular with large followings during their lifetime. They had many commonalities yet, they never met. They had an influence on the populations of two countries, the United States and Mexico. Both Don Pedrito and Teresita were born in Mexico but lived and had many patients in the United States, and Niño Fidencio still has a large following of Fidencista believers not only in Mexico but also throughout the United States.

We also learned about four, ***Curanderos(as) of Recent Times: Impacting the United States and Mexico,*** who have passed on but also had an impact on *curanderismo* in the United States and Mexico. They also had some commonalities including publications and having had some articles written about them.

Just like the *curanderos* of yesteryear and those of recent times, the following section highlights several *curanderos(as)* from Mexico and the United States that have contributed and impacted traditional medicine in two countries through their rituals, therapies, mentoring, and teachings. We will discover how many of these talented *curanderos(as)* are well trained in modern allopathic medicine, as well as traditional medicine and are developing a new health model to meet the needs of many of our citizens from both countries, just like the final group of young professionals are doing in the last section of this publication called ***Curanderos(as) of Tomorrow***. The reader can learn about these healers in a brief biography, as well as in the captions describing the photos.

The first *curandero* is called a *materia,* which is the title that the *Fidencista* followers use in describing Cresencio Alvarado Nuñez, known as Chenchito, a healer who has impacted the lives of hundreds in Mexico and the United States. He lives on the Mexican–Texas border and frequently crosses to the American side to see patients and friends. Recently, at the age of 90, he came to the University of New Mexico to share his wisdom and perform his magical healings with the students and community. Chenchito has been my mentor and teacher for almost 30 years.

I have known Rita Navarrete for almost 20 years when she and several *curanderos(as)* traveled 20 hours by bus from the Mexico City area to the University of New Mexico for an International Conference on Traditional Medicine. This multi-talented *curandera* has presented many class sessions for the summer course, as well as the online classes, on a number of topics such as medicinal plants, fire cupping/*ventosas*, shawl alignments/*manteadas*, Laugh Therapy/*Risa Terapia*, water therapy/*hidroterapia*, sweat lodge/*temazcal*, and many others. She has also seen hundreds of patients from throughout Mexico and the United States.

Toñita Gonzales is a protege of Rita Navarrete. They met at a workshop, Rita was conducting in Albuquerque on Laugh Therapy, and Rita invited Toñita to Mexico City to train with her and to attend Dr. Ornelas' holistic medicine school in Cuernavaca. After two years, Toñita received her diploma from the school and returned to New Mexico. She opened a clinic with a *temazcal* sweat lodge in the North Valley of Albuquerque. She has treated a number of patients from all throughout the United States and lectures internationally to a number of groups including medical students and physicians. Having studied and lived in Mexico City, Toñita is a unique healer that is proficient in two cultures and two languages and is now teaching her skills to a number of individuals interning under her guidance.

Maclovia Sánchez de Zamora is a well-known herbalist who continues serving the community of Albuquerque and has been featured in a number of articles for her contributions to the lives of New Mexicans. She has a popular herb store called Ruppe Drugs.

I have known Laura Alonzo de Franklin for almost 20 years, since she was an apprentice of the late *curandera* Elena Avila. She has studied traditional medicine in Cuernavaca and Oaxaca, Mexico. She is referred to as Maestra/ Teacher Laura, has a *temazcal* sweat lodge, and has mentored a large number of students from throughout the country under the auspices of a community sacred house called Kalpulli Teocalli Ollin.

Two healers from Mexico who come from a lineage of *curanderos(as)* and have certain specialties are Agustin Pérez, *huesero*/bonesetter from Mexico City and Laurencio Nuñez a *temazcalero*/sweat lodge guide from Oaxaca, Mexico, who recently relocated to Puebla, Mexico.

There are three other healers who are from different parts of the country and are committed to traditional healing and continue incorporating this practice into their professions. Bob Vetter, an anthropologist from New York, has blended *curanderismo* into the spirituality and healing of the Southern Plains tribes. Alex Jackson from Kansas City, Missouri, has specialized in Mayan Abdominal Massage, while Kim Hart from Minneapolis, Minnesota, has developed the Adagio Holistic Therapies clinic and incorporates traditional methods in her treatments.

Marcia Valdez from northern New Mexico has been practicing traditional medicine for 30 years and Katherine White, who lives in Albuquerque, retired after almost 30 years as a registered nurse to become an expert herbalist specializing in medicinal plants and *curanderismo*.

Dr. Arturo Ornelas, Director and President of the Center for Community Human Development School, has an impressive faculty well prepared to teach a number of traditional therapies. In addition to their instruction, they are practitioners with many of them directing their own health clinics in different Mexican communities. Many of these healers can trace their ancestors to lineages of *curanderos(as)* and they are the only health providers of their small rural communities. They are proficient in a number of traditional therapies that are evident in the photos, captions, and biographies you will enjoy in this section. These faculty/*curanderos(as)* are Rita Navarrete, Velia Herrera, Tana Sánchez, Lety Amaro, and Doris Ortiz. Other practicing *curanderos(as)* are Maria Nely Mancillas, Daniel Duran, Maria del Carmen Ayala, Carmen Ramírez, Maria Lucia Flores, and Toñita Gonzales.

In the final group, three have PhDs with their doctorates in a number of fields, doctors and clergy. All have incorporated *curanderismo* into their profession creating a new health model. The PhDs are Drs. Tomas Enos from Santa Fe, New Mexico, Ysamur Flores from Los Angeles, California, and Felina Ortiz from Albuquerque, New Mexico. Selma Sroka from Minneapolis, Minnesota, is a medical doctor and the Reverend Virginia Marie Rincón an Episcopal priest who recently relocated from Texas to New Mexico.

In *Curanderos(as)* **of Nowadays: Creating a New Traditional Healing Model,** you will be able to learn and enjoy a number of photos about the healers who are committed to serving their community with a new healing model and teaching others preventive medicine and therapies that are effective and easy to learn.

CRESENCIO ALVARADO NUŃEZ AKA "CHENCHITO"

Chenchito is a name of endearment that is appropriate for a kind and gentle person who has touched the lives of hundreds of people in the United States and Mexico. He has a home in the town of Control, Tamaulipas, Mexico, and a second one in Espinazo, Nuevo León, Mexico, a small village where the famous Niño Fidencio lived and died in 1938. Chenchito has been a *curandero* all of his life and is called a *materia* or medium, which is the term used for healers that follow the Fidencista movement, considered a folk religion by many. At times, Chenchito channels the spirit of El Niño Fidencio in order to perform his healings. He is one of the last *materias* who met one of Mexico's most famous healers and is still living as of the publication of this book.

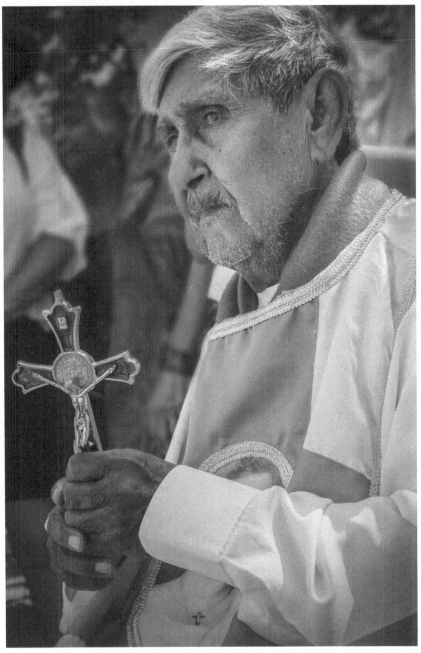

Chenchito blesses an opening ceremony for a community healing event in Santa Fe, New Mexico. Chenchito and other healers provided a variety of healing sessions to the public including spiritual cleansings, massages, and fire cupping. Chenchito wears a white and a purple vestment, similar to that of a priest, containing an image of El Niño Fidencio. He invoked the spirit of El Niño and called upon God to bless the ceremony. As a spiritual healer, Chenchito uses the Christian Cross and holy water in a way that merges traditional rituals with recognized religion.

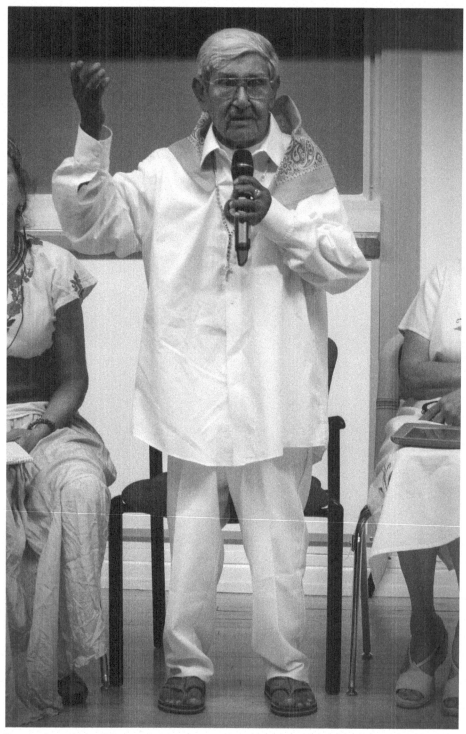

Chenchito gives a talk to students of the University of New Mexico *curanderismo* course about his devotion to the Fidencista movement. He explained that it is arduous work and requires serious commitment. At the age of almost 90 years old, he and one assistant made a 900 mile road trip to participate in the course. They traveled from the town of Control, Tamaulipas, Mexico, to Albuquerque, New Mexico. During the trip, the vehicle in which they traveled suffered an accident. Despite the hardships, Chenchito arrived safely. He believes that this tragic incident was a sign from the spirit of Niño Fidencio that tested his faith.

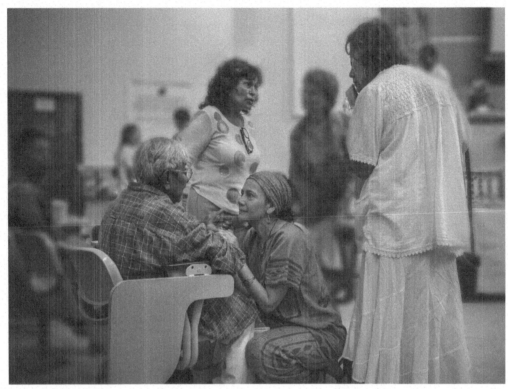

Some students of the *curanderismo* course at the University of New Mexico were eager to meet Chenchito, ask questions, and receive blessings. Chenchito has touched the lives and hearts of many people in Mexico and the Southwest.

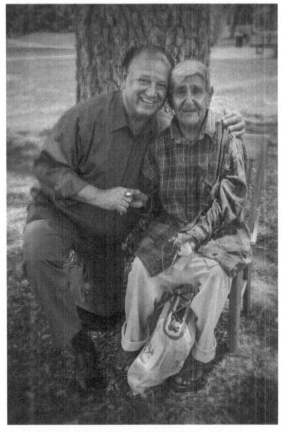

Dr. Eliseo "Cheo" Torres poses for a photograph with Chenchito after completing his lecture at the traditional medicine course at the University of New Mexico. Chenchito has known Cheo for 30 years and has been his teacher and mentor.

RITA NAVARRETE

Rita has been an instructor at the traditional medicine summer school for almost 20 years. Rita is a *curandera*, *temazcalera*, *sobadora*, *consejera*, *yerbera*, *quiropractico*/traditional chiropractor, and a motivational speaker. This multi-talented healer has practiced traditional healing for over 32 years and directs a traditional medicine center in Mataxhi, Mexico, and a health clinic in Mexico City. Some of the classes that she teaches include sweat lodges, massage, fire cupping, laugh therapy, and medicinal plants, as well as supporting and assisting survivors of domestic violence. She has been a presenter at the Smithsonian Institute in Washington, D.C. and several cities throughout the United States.

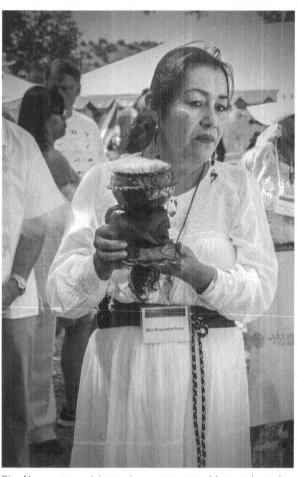

Rita Navarrete participates in a ceremony to bless and smudge a public health fair using *copal* incense in Santa Fe, New Mexico.

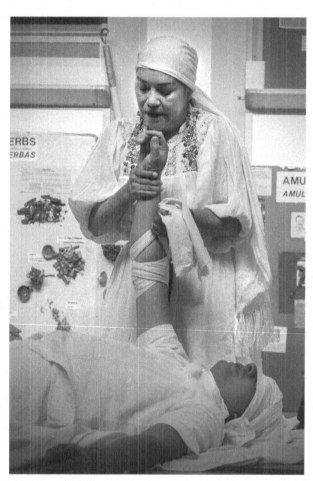

Rita Navarrete demonstrates a healing body adjustment practice involving the muscular and skeletal system during the *curanderismo* course at the University of New Mexico. Rita uses unbleached cotton material to demonstrate the practice called shawl alignments referred to as *manteadas* in Mexico.

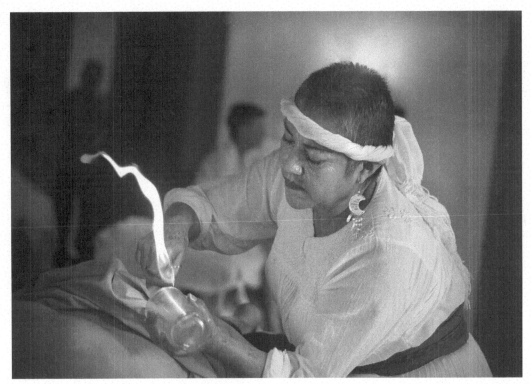

Rita Navarrete uses fire cupping, known as *ventosas* in Mexico, on a patient. Rita treated several people using this method at a public traditional health fair hosted at the National Hispanic Cultural Center in Albuquerque. *Ventosas* warm muscles and improve blood circulation to help patients suffering from cervical, sciatic, and lumbar problems.

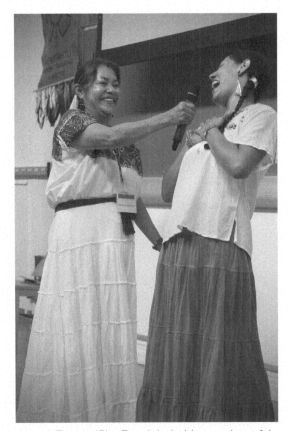

Rita Navarrete demonstrates the use of Laugh Therapy/*Risa Terapia* by inviting members of the *curanderismo* class to step up to the podium and laugh in various ways.

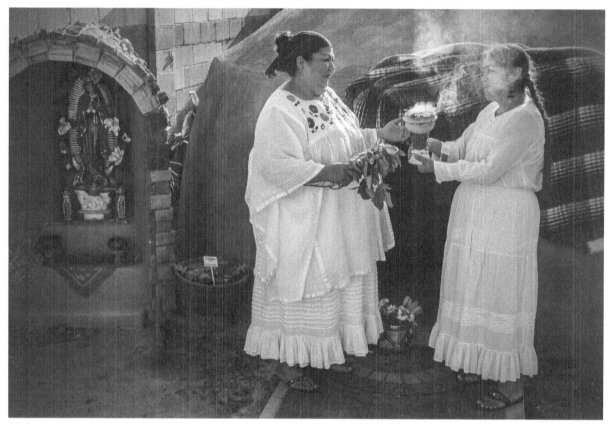

Toñita Gonzales (left) and Rita Navarrete (right) stand in front of *Temazcal Tonantzin*, a sweat lodge located in the North Valley of Albuquerque. Toñita holds a branch of Basil *Albahaca/Ocimum basilicum* and Rita an incense burner called *sahumerio* or *popoxcomitl*, commonly used with *copal* incense in Mexican sweat lodge ceremonies. An altar dedicated to the Virgin of Guadalupe connects the sweat lodge practice with its Mexican and indigenous roots.

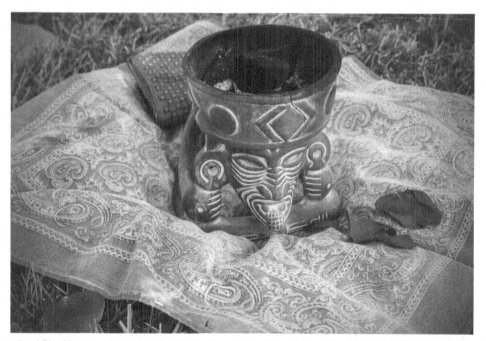

The picture above is of Rita Navarrete's *sahumerio* with the face of the Aztec God of Fire, Xiuhtecuhtli, which she uses in *limpias*, prayers, and ceremonies. The incense burner represents the sacred union between the physical and the spiritual worlds. Healers send their intentions to the cosmos using *copal* incense smoke as a channel. The smoke also symbolizes a union between the Earth and the Sky, which according to healers, creates a sacred equilibrium.

TOÑITA GONZALES

Toñita Gonzales is a native of New Mexico. Her family is from Gonzales Ranch, which is located 55 miles southeast of Santa Fe, New Mexico, and is proud of her blending of cultures which allows her to serve a diverse community. She studied traditional medicine at the Center for Community Human Development mentioned in chapter one.

Toñita works with the community in Albuquerque and northern New Mexico to provide traditional medicine treatments and education on the medicine of the ancestors.

After two years of classes in Cuernavaca and an internship in Mexico City with her mentor and teacher, Rita Navarrete, Toñita has become a nationally renowned healer and speaker. She began her practice in the Mexican community of Mataxhi where she and Rita Navarrete organized a health clinic and outreach center. She has a clinic and a *temazcal* in the North Valley of Albuquerque that serves a large number of clients from the community, students, and allied health professionals. She is the founder and director of RAICES (Remembering Ancestors, Inspiring Community, and Empowering Self), an organization that draws on ancient wisdom to provide traditional medicine education to the community of New Mexico and beyond.

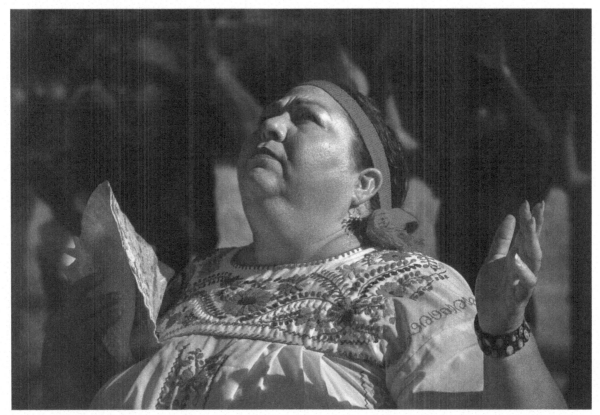

Toñita Gonzales holds a conch shell horn (called an *atecocolli* in the Nahuatl language or *caracol* in Spanish) used during a ceremony that honors the four directions, the Mother Earth and the Father Sky. The seashell is typically used in such ceremonies to represent wind and water. Along with the use of rattles, drums, and other tools, it is blown to call the healing energies for guidance.

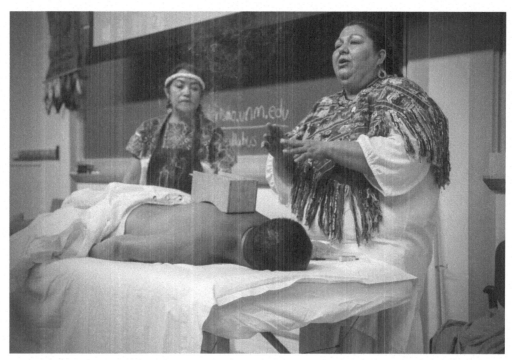

Toñita Gonzales teaches a class with her mentor Rita Navarrete at the *curanderismo* class at the University of New Mexico. Toñita demonstrates the use of a moxibustion box, which is also used in traditional Chinese medicine. The demonstration consisted of burning dried mugwort leaves/*Estafiate*/*Ocimum basilicum* near the skin to treat shoulder pain.

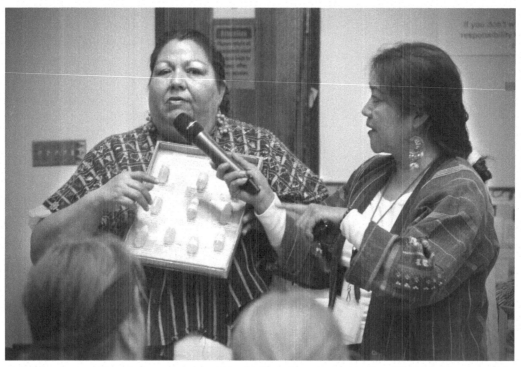

Toñita Gonzales gives a presentation on tinctures used to help the digestive system and relieve high blood pressure during the *curanderismo* course at the University of New Mexico. Toñita has extensive experience lecturing on traditional medicine. Her knowledge of traditional medicine in English and Spanish allows her to quickly interpret terms for her audience from one language to the other.

LAURENCIO NUÑEZ

Laurencio is a native of Oaxaca, Mexico. He started his journey in *curanderismo* at the age of six. He credits his grandmother for her teaching and inspiration. He reports to have had visions, which led him to become a *curandero*. This gentle and kind healer was trained as a botanist and became a healer specializing in *limpias*, medicinal herbology, and the *temazcal*. He has worked with marginalized communities in rural areas of Oaxaca, Mexico, and has recently relocated to Puebla, Mexico. Laurencio is a regular instructor in the summer *curanderismo* class as well as in the online course.

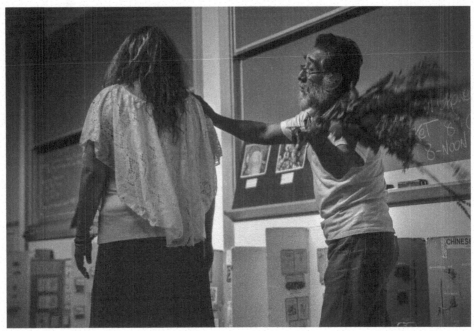

Laurencio Nuñez uses a bundle of aromatic plants to do a spiritual cleanse/*limpia* during the *curanderismo* class. In this image, he uses Lavender/*Alhucema/Lavandula sp.*, Rosemary/Romero/*Rosmarinus officinalis*, and Basil/*Albahaca/Ocimum basilicum* in addition to other tools to perform the cleansing. Laurencio blesses the plants and asks for divine permission before beginning.

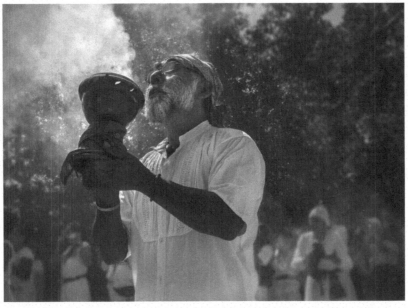

Laurencio Nuñez blows into a *sahumerio* filled with burning charcoal and *copal* incense, which are typically used for ceremonies and *limpias*. Here, Laurencio participates in a ceremony to bless a public health fair in Santa Fe, New Mexico.

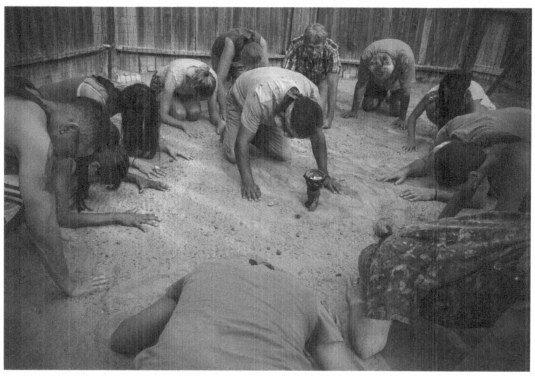

Laurencio Nuñez leads a ceremony honoring the four directions, the Mother Earth and the Father Sky. He conducts ceremonies like these to prepare groups to enter *temazcal* sessions. In this image, Laurencio prepares a group in Los Lunas, New Mexico.

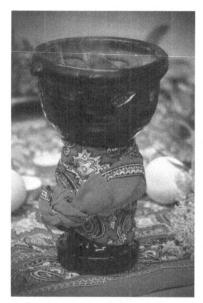

Pictured above is the incense burner used by Laurencio for spiritual cleansings. In addition, Laurencio uses fresh herbs, eggs, candles, and red kerchiefs called *paliacates* as tools during the cleansings her performs.

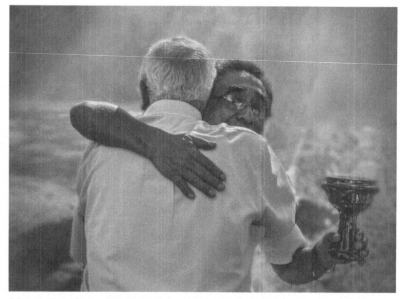

After performing a spiritual cleansing, Laurencio Nuñez embraces the recipient as a gesture of compassion. Laurencio begins each *limpia* by asking questions and carefully listening to his patients. He uses listening and embracing as part of the healing practice and a means to express kinship.

VELIA HERRERA

Velia is a healer in her village outside of the historical town of Tepoztlan, Mexico. She is an instructor of holistic medicine at the Center for Community Human Development, specializing in *limpias* and other traditional healing therapies. She also performs massage and healing with medicinal plants. Velia has her own consultation clinic in Central Mexico.

She identifies herself as a native traditional healer who treats patients using the elements of nature that her native culture still practices with such as rocks, small animals, plants, and other tools not commonly associated with allopathic medicine. She works closely with sacred energies and performs a ceremony to find spiritual guidance.

Velia would be described by the late healer Elena Avila in her book, "**Woman Who Glows in the Dark**" as an *Espiritualista*/Spiritualist healer. Such healers can go into a trance in order to create a conduit between the spiritual and the material realms. Other *curanderos(as)* that have this gift are Chenchito and Felipa, described earlier in this book.

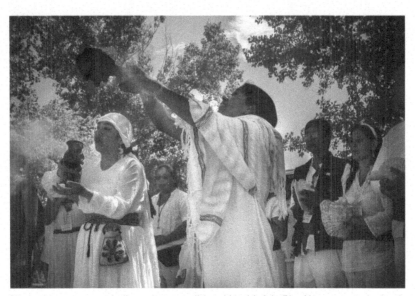

Velia honors the Father Sky in this ceremony dedicated to a traditional health fair. Rita Navarrete and other healers are using symbolic objects to greet and honor the directions of the East with the conch shell horn, West with the drums, South with the rattles, and North with the whistles. Each direction is honored separately and all participants turn, kneel, or look up accordingly.

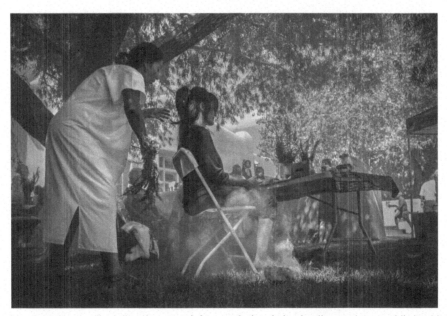

Velia calls the energies of the four cardinal directions to ask for permission do her healing work at a public health fair in Santa Fe, New Mexico.

According to Velia, in honoring the four directions, the direction of the East represents rebirth; the West represents the energy of the night wind; the North represents the energy of the grandparents, as well as relaxation and rest; and the South represents the warrior energy associated with the humming bird/*colibri*. It should be noted that each healer and culture has their own interpretation of the four directions.

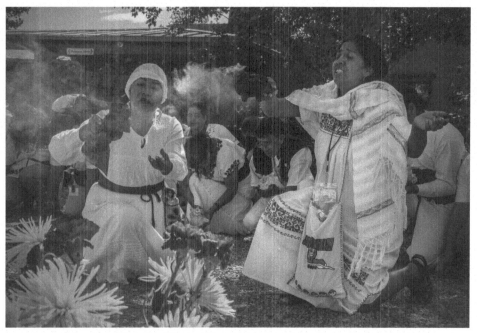

In this ceremony, healers evoke the energies of the Mother Earth, Father Sun, and the four directions as preparation for their work. Velia Herrera (right), Rita Navarrete (left), and other healers kneel to honor the sacred energy of Mother Earth before offering healing sessions at a public health fair in Santa Fe, New Mexico.

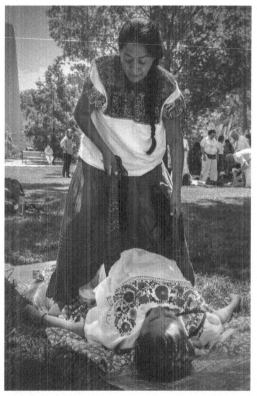

Velia demonstrates a *manteada* utilized to align the hips. The technique is used to relieve problems caused by bad posture, lifting heavy objects, and postpartum stress. *Manteadas* are effective with pregnant women, children, and the elderly.

ALBERTANA SÁNCHEZ

Albertana is known as Tana and has several diplomas in traditional and integrated medicine such as the preparation of tinctures and microdosages using medicinal plants, holistic massage, oriental massages, Aztec flowers for healing, and biomagnetism. Tana teaches and serves patients in the clinic connected to the Center for Community Human Development institute and school. Her speciality is addressing a number of chronic illnesses. Tana has been a regular instructor at the annual summer school at the University of New Mexico and has done a video for the online class on *empacho*.

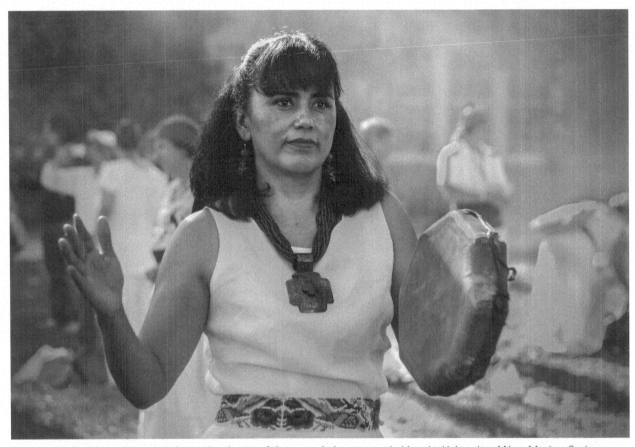

Tana uses a drum in a ceremony to honor the closure of the *curanderismo* course held at the University of New Mexico. Such ceremonies are offered to the students, healers, and the larger community that participates in this course. Through the vibrations of the drums, the aroma of *copal* incense, and the sound of the sea shell conch/*atecocolli*, the healers honor the four directions and the elements earth, wind, fire, and water. These elements are important to healers because they help them call the sacred energies that guide them in their practice.

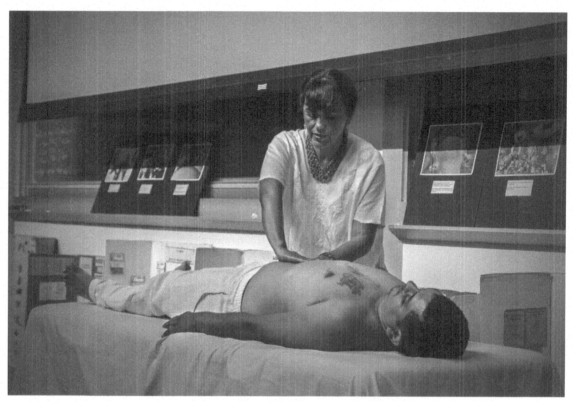

Tana demonstrates a technique to relieve *empacho* that involves massaging the patient's abdomen and lower back while pulling on the skin in order to dislodge the blockage. Tana is a regular presenter at University of New Mexico's *curanderismo* class.

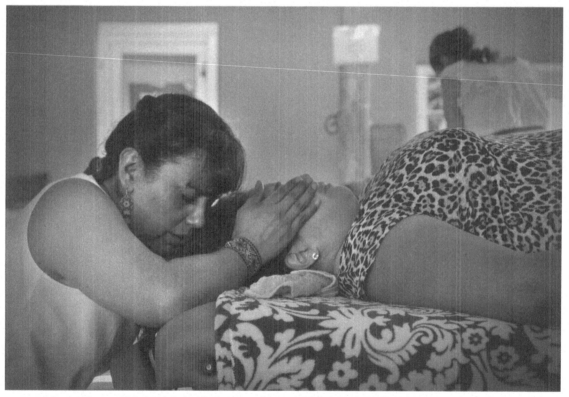

Tana treats a patient with stressful emotions by singing a soothing song for a gentle healing session. According to her, such emotions impact the body in the form of depression, anxiety, and problems with the digestive system.

MARIA ADORACIÓN ORTIZ

Maria Adoración, known as Doris, learned the skills of *curanderismo* from her grandmother who was her teacher for more than 20 years, especially in the area of medicinal plants. She is an instructor in the traditional medicine school in Cuernavaca and she has several diplomas including psychotherapy, naturopathy, and acupuncture. Her strength is on medicinal plants, knowing their healing properties as well as their common and scientific names. She uses medicinal plants in preparing alcohol-based tinctures and water-based microdosages, cough syrups, ointments, and oils, and prescribes them in her traditional health clinic.

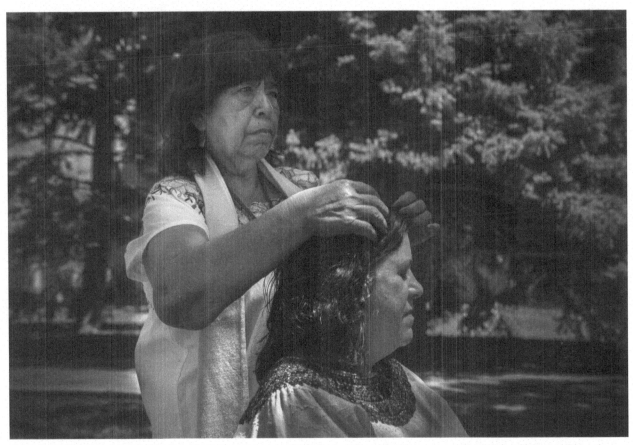

Maria Adoración is known as Maestra Doris. In this image, she balances the patient's energy so that it flows from a position of stagnation to one of healing activity through meridians that flow from the head to the feet. She uses energy from her hands to stabilize emotions and dispel negative ones. In this image, Maestra Doris is a participant of a traditional medicine health fair that was held at the University of New Mexico.

MARCIA VALDEZ, LMT

Marcia Valdez grew up in the mountainous area of Vadito, New Mexico. Her goal has always been to serve humanity through the healing arts. Her gentle approach focuses on awareness of our place in the cosmos and the belief that healers act as conduits between the sacred healing energies and the patient.

Marcia studied with Mary Burmeister, one of the foremost teachers of Jin Shin Jyutsu, which is a Japanese healing art with ancient roots. She studied with naturopathic doctor Robin Murphy and with the late Elena Avila briefly. She continues to study with Rita Navarrete and Toñita Gonzales.

Marcia embraces a humble attitude toward traditional medicine. Some refer to her as a *curandera,* but she prefers the title of health facilitator. She has lived and practiced traditional medicine in Santa Fe, New Mexico for over 30 years and maintained a clinic in the same location for 20 years. She calls her practice body wisdom because she listens to her hands and the spirit of her patients as she works on them. Her practice often involves energy work, deep tissue massage, *limpias*, and at times counseling conversations/*platicas*.

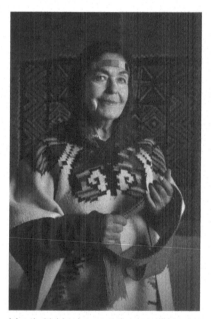

Marcia Valdez has practiced traditional medicine for over 30 years in Santa Fe, New Mexico. She holds a type of red sash that is commonly used in traditional healing to protect practitioners from negative energies.

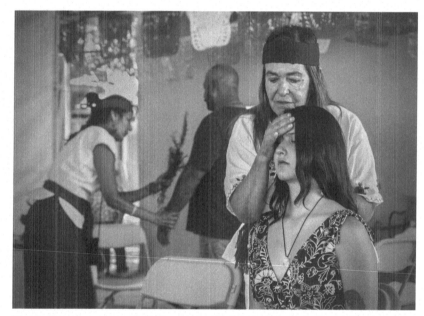

Marcia uses stones, a sage plant, and breathing techniques to help a patient at a health fair in Santa Fe, New Mexico. She often reminds people not to hold their breath and to breathe properly in order to optimize the healing process.

LAURA ALONZO DE FRANKLIN, MSW, PHD CANDIDATE

Laura Alonzo de Franklin (Cuauhtli Cihuatl) is a *curandera*, spiritual healer, community advocate, and health promoter who has worked in New Mexico for 35 years. She was born in San Benito, Texas, but raised in Tampico, Mexico, with her grandmother Casimira Rocha Sánchez, a *curandera*. She is commonly known as Maestra CC or the "Rock & Roll *Curandera*" for her musical endeavors. She grew up with Freddy Fender's music and a passion for Stevie Ray Vaughn music. A local musician from New Mexico, Paul Pino, wrote and recorded the "Rock & Roll *Curandera*" for her.

As an empath, intuitive, and traditional healer, she uses clinical social work methods and evidence-based practices including indigenous ceremonies, heart-to-heart talks *platicas*, *sweat lodges*, prayer, meditation, herbal consultations, soul retrievals among other practices. She does energy work for the immigrant community, incarcerated Native American youth, veterans, young mothers, hospice patients, and those in addiction recovery. Much of her work focuses on helping returning Afghanistan and Iraq veterans cope with *susto* or PTSD.

Laura performs cross-cultural spiritual practices and is initiated into the Mexhika, Aztec, Lipan Apache, and Lakota traditions as a medicine woman. She has been the guardian of a Mexhika *temazcal* for the past 11 ps built on her home in Los Lunas, New Mexico. She founded Kalpulli Teocalli Ollin in 2004, an indigenous community of teaching, learning, and offering traditional healing to the community, which includes apprentices from twelve states. Maestra CC continues to carry the medicine as her *abuelita* Casimira taught her *"la medicina es para todos"*/the medicine is for all.

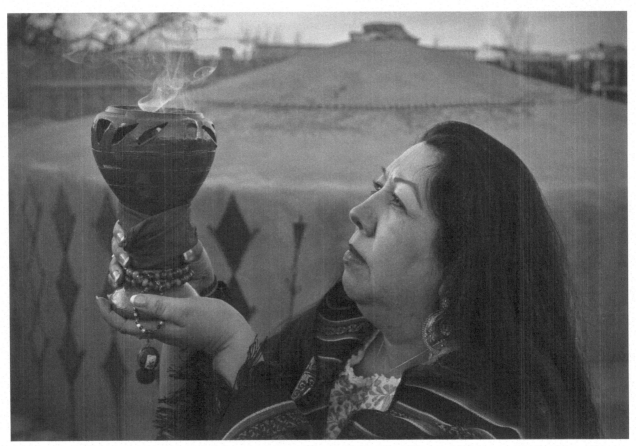

Maestra Laura holds her *sahumerio* in Los Lunas, New Mexico. Pictured behind her is Temazcal Ollin, a sweat lodge directed by Maestra Laura where has led many healing sessions.

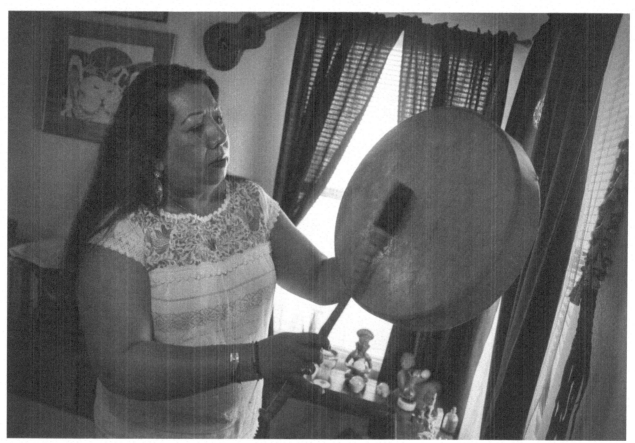

Maestra Laura uses various tools for healing purposes. As a multicultural healer, she draws from various sources including Lipan Apache and Mexican traditions as well as her training as a social worker. At her place of healing, she keeps a collection of drums, Mesoamerican inspired statuettes, and musical instruments.

DR. TOMAS ENOS

Before receiving his PhD for his research on *curanderismo* and holistic healing, Dr. Tomas Enos completed a two-year apprenticeship and study of traditional healing practices in Oaxaca, Mexico. He is now the president and owner of Milagro Herbs in Santa Fe, New Mexico. As an ethnobotanist, he prepares a number of herbal products and teaches several classes on the identification and preparation of medicinal plants. He continues practicing a holistic approach to healing body, mind, and spirit through applications of herbal medicine, counseling, reflexology, and visualization techniques. He is a regular presenter at the two-week curanderismo class and the online course at the University of New Mexico.

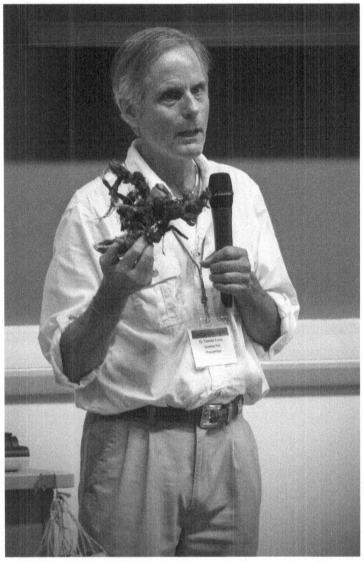

Dr. Tomas Enos speaks to the students of the traditional medicine class at the University of New Mexico. Dr. Enos stressed the importance of using medicinal herbs and plants to provide holistic healing.

He explained that by using allopathic medicine, with the approval of your physician, in conjunction with herbs and plants, it is possible to create an effective form of integrated medicine. In this image, he holds one of the most popular herbs that grows in the mountains of Albuquerque, the osha root/*chuchupate,* and discusses its various medicinal properties and applications, especially for the respiratory system.

VIRIDIANA MEDINA

Viridiana is referred to as Viri and collaborates with another well-known healer, Juan Carlos, who is described in this publication. Viri supports him in serving several Mexican rural communities with traditional health services. She leads several groups in a *temazcal* connected to their clinic, Kalpulli Ome, located in the small community of Huitzilac, Morelos, Mexico. The word Kalpulli is used to describe a sacred house of healing or a community group formed to promote traditions, history and dance. Many of the Mexican *temazcales* have titles with Nahuatl (Aztec) language names beginning with the word *kalpulli*, meaning "community." Viri has attended, participated, and taught at the annual summer *curanderismo* class and specializes in a number of traditional healing therapies, especially *limpias*.

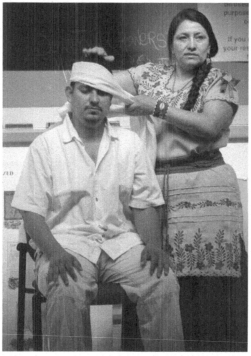

Viri demonstrates the application of shawl alignments for injuries resulting from accidents. She mentioned that it is helpful to press the body with a shawl/*manta* after receiving an impact so that the body can recover its equilibrium.

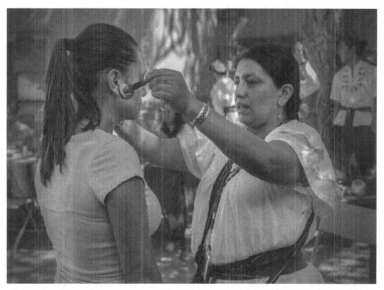

Viri performs a *limpia* using rattles and *copal* incense at a public health fair in Santa Fe, New Mexico. According to Viri, the vibrations and the *copal* aroma can harmonize the patient's emotions, energy, and spirit thereby recovering clarity and awareness.

JUAN CARLOS SOLANO

Juan Carlos is a well-known healer that has connected the Mesoamerican cosmovision of understanding the world's view of time and space to *curanderismo*. His Aztec name is *Xihuacatl* and one of his healing specialties is using the vibrational sound of the conch shell horn/*caracol* or *atecocolli* in the Nahuatl language in combination with the volcanic smooth and shiny obsidian stone. He uses both elements of the conch shell horn and obsidian stone to perform his intensive *limpias* also called *tonalli* cleansing. He connects the conch shell horn to the Aztec mythical God, *Quetzalcoatl*, the feathered serpent who brings clarity and wisdom to the patient. The black mirror-like obsidian stone is correlated to a second Aztec God, brother of *Quetzalcoatl*, *Tezcatlipoca*, whose name means "Smoky Mirror" and is connected to our ancestors. In this *limpia*, the conch shell horn sound creates vibrations surrounds the patient in order to bring clarity and wisdom while the obsidian stone is carefully placed on the naval area of the stomach in order to allow the ancestors to help with the healing process.

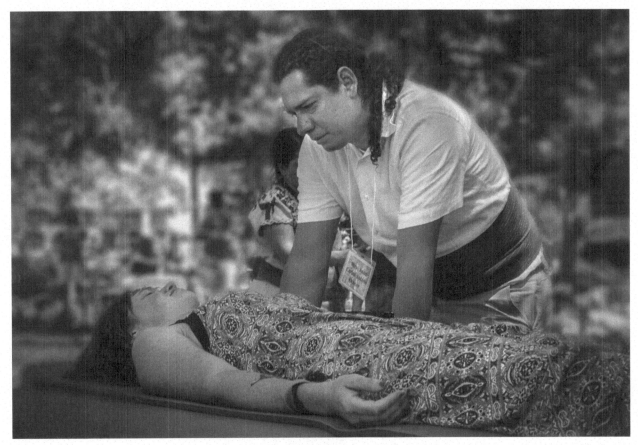

Juan Carlos listens attentively to the concerns and stories of his patient during a health fair held at the University of New Mexico. Traditional healers often start a healing practice by listening to the patient for several minutes to determine the proper treatment.

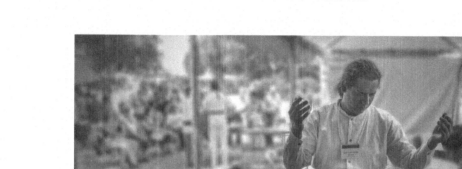

Juan Carlos performs a treatment using obsidian stones placed on the naval area in combination with the vibrational sounds of the conch shell horn. According to Juan Carlos when we use these tools, not only we can bring healing to the body, but also we can tune into the harmony of the universe.

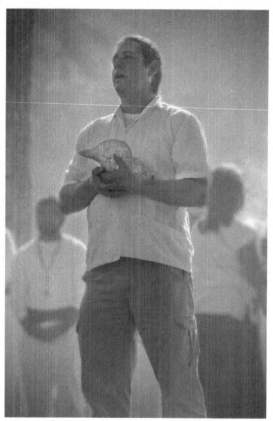

Juan Carlos leads a ceremony at the University of New Mexico that uses conch shell horns/*caracoles*, drums, incense burners, and rattles/*sonajas* to symbolize earth, wind, fire, and water. When these elements come together in the ceremony, according to Juan Carlos, a microcosm is created allowing practitioners to connect with healing energy and find guidance.

MARIA NELY MANCILLA

Maria Nely is referred to as Nely and comes from a lineage of healers and herbalists. Her mother was a midwife for the town of Olinalá, in the state of Guerrero, Mexico. Her brother, grandmother, and great grandmother were *curanderos(as)*.

At the age of nine, Nely's family started training her in traditional healing. At that age she was old enough to assist her mother to obtain her midwifery certification. Because her mother did not know how to write, Nely took notes on obstetrics. Experiencing firsthand the tradition of midwifery, she assisted her mother in providing *manteadas* to pregnant women. With the help of this training, at the age of 16, Nely delivered her first baby because her mother was out of town.

She recalls how her high school classmates came to her for sports injuries because the school did not have a nurse on staff. On one occasion, she assisted a classmate with a dislocated ankle. She learned from her mother and brother massage therapies and bone setting.

Her love of plants is evident in her lush garden of medicinal plants located at her home in Cuernavaca, considered the "City of Eternal Spring"/"*La Ciudad de la Eterna Primavera*" since its climate is ideal, year-round, for growing plants and flowers. This environment may be the reason why Nely became an herbalist/*yerbera*. In her work, she grows her plants and flowers and makes her own medicinal tinctures. A second specialty of Nely is that of being a *sobadora* combined with body adjustments and as practiced by *hueseros*.

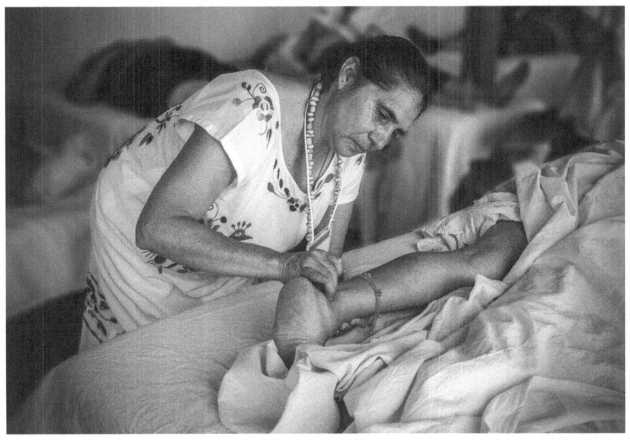

Nely stimulates, through acupressure, the kidney and bladder channels to relieve the patient from stagnation and allow a better flow of energy. According to her, this massage allows the patient to release negative emotions, like fear, once he/she has relaxed. Santa Fe, New Mexico.

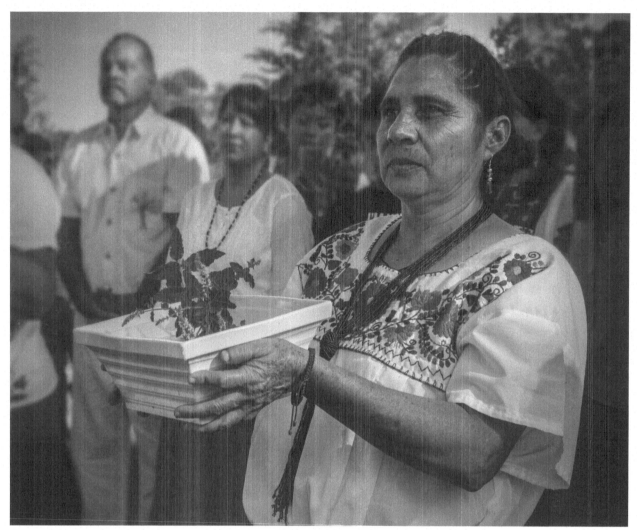

Nely has a deep connection with plants. At her home in Cuernavaca, she maintains a garden where she grows lime trees, colorful flowers, chiles, berries, aloe vera, and various medicinal plants. In this image, she holds a plant at the University of New Mexico to demonstrate the importance of Mother Earth in traditional healing.

LETICIA AMARO

Leticia is known as Lety and has been practicing and teaching traditional medicine for several years. She is an instructor at the Center of Community Human Development in Mexico and an instructor in the *curanderismo* class in New Mexico. She teaches and practices traditional *sobadas*, *limpias*, Mayan acupuncture, and other modalities of healing. One of her specialties is plants for the nervous system and Lety states, "mother nature gives us exceptional plants that help with the nervous system so that our body continues to work the way it needs to." Some of the plants that she recommends for the nervous system are as follows: Lavender/*Alucema*, Rosemary/*Romero*, Passion Flower/*Passiflora*. Lety uses medicinal plants with *limpias* for a more effective therapy in addressing the nervous system.

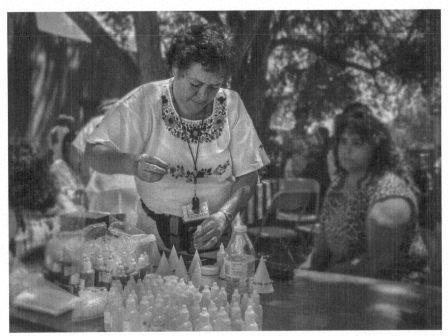

Lety prepares a water-based microdosage (similar to homeopathic medicine) for a patient at a traditional medicine health fair in Santa Fe, New Mexico.

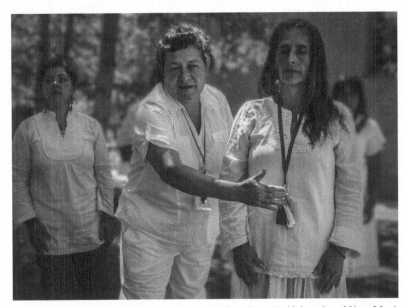

Lety teaches a way to perceive the energy of another person using the hands at the University of New Mexico. This technique involves moving the hands slowly and closely through the body of another person to detect subtle sensations. With practice, one can become sensitive to detect pain according to Lety. She calls it, "the human x-ray."

DANIEL DURAN

Daniel Duran grew up in Santa Maria, Tonanitla, a village located 20 miles north of Mexico City. The name of the village, according to Daniel, has its roots in *Tonantzin*, which is Mother Earth in Aztec mythology. To this day, he lives and has his clinic in this village, which he refers to as "the place where the Mother Earth is venerated."

At the age of 16, Daniel received a prediction from his uncle that he would help people heal. Intrigued by the remarks, Daniel began learning about traditional medicine on his own but realized that he needed guidance and eventually attended the University of Chapingo in Central Mexico where he learned to appreciate the knowledge of his indigenous ancestors and the natural world.

Daniel has a profound awareness of the natural and spiritual worlds. At a public health fair, he helped a college student relieve stress by instructing him to place his hands on a tree for a few minutes in a meditative-like session to do breathing exercises. According to Daniel, the tree helped discharge the student's negative energy and moved it toward the earth, thereby burying it. He recognizes that plants, trees, and sunlight have a considerable impact in our lives.

Daniel is soft-spoken, gentle, and a good listener. He enjoys teaching his knowledge of the human body to those willing to learn. To him, teaching is like planting a seed that will grow and bloom.

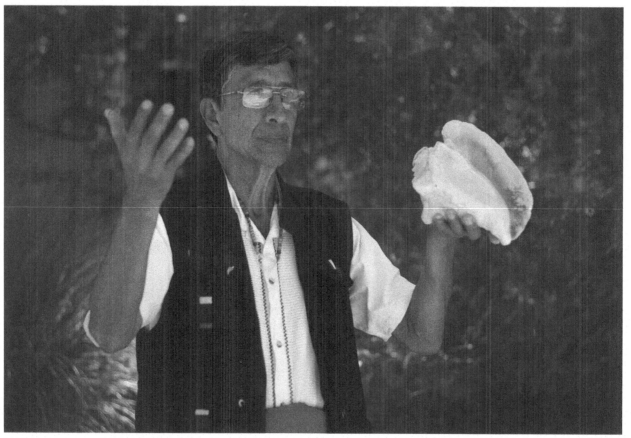

Daniel holds a conch shell horn that he uses during ceremonies dedicated to the four directions and the elements of earth, wind, fire, and water at the University of New Mexico.

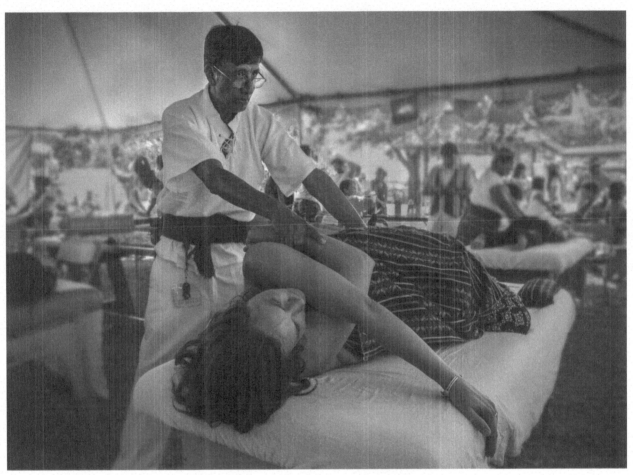

Daniel relieves a woman from back pain by slowly pressing the muscles located along the spinal cord starting from the cervical area and concluding at the lumbar section. In addition, he massages the patient's lower back and instructs her to stretch her arms as part of the therapy.

MARIA DEL CARMEN AYALA AND CARMEN RAMÍREZ

Maria del Carmen Ayala and Carmen Ramírez both live in Mexico City but in distinct neighborhoods. Both run their own practices but when they visit Albuquerque to participate in the traditional medicine summer course, they always work together. According to Maria, by working together, they are able to treat patients in a more effective manner because their energies as healers synchronize well.

Maria believes that she was born to practice traditional medicine. In Mexico and in the Southwest people, use the phrase "*tiene el don*" to refer to the condition of a person who is "gifted" in a certain profession or skill. Maria believes that some people have "the unique gift" to help others heal and that she has the gift.

According to her, a great majority of ailments are psychosomatic in nature. That is, they are illnesses that are caused or worsened by mental factors. She specializes in working with people's emotions and has helped many with bipolar disorder and strong emotions. In addition, she has helped people suffering from paralysis, heart attacks, psoriasis, and cancer.

Carmen started in 2009 when searching for a personal healing. After receiving several therapies, she became fond of traditional medicine and wanted to pursue training. She studied under Maria and both developed a close friendship. Carmen agrees with her teacher that the great majority of people's problems come from their emotions. Both believe that each person deserves a unique treatment because each one of us is different.

Both specialize in energetic massage, acupuncture, osteopathy, chiropractic, and energy work. Their introduction to traditional medicine began because they both wanted to heal at personal levels.

In Mexico, people typically refer to Maria and Carmen as therapists and doctors but according to Maria, she has never claimed to be a doctor. She has working relations with doctors and has treated some of them. She believes that doctors have a scientific, step-by-step approach with their patients, while the therapist employs intuition, love, and compassion and learns to read body and face language, to diagnose through looking at the tongue, and even the belly button, in order to identify problems.

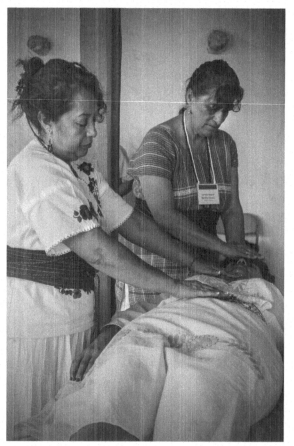

Maria del Carmen Ayala (right) and her colleague Carmen Ramírez (left) conclude a Reiki therapy by aligning the chakra points of their patient, Albertana Sánchez. Healers also benefit from receiving treatment from their colleagues as this image illustrates. At the start of this health fair and at its conclusion, healers take breaks to receive treatments.

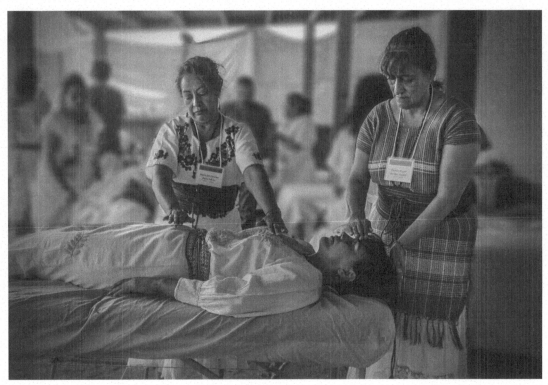

Maria del Carmen Ayala (right) and her colleague Carmen Ramírez (left) conduct the Reiki therapy illustrated on a previous page. This session did not involve touch. According to Maria del Carmen, by hovering their hands over the patient's body, they were able to better assist the patient. Santa Fe, New Mexico.

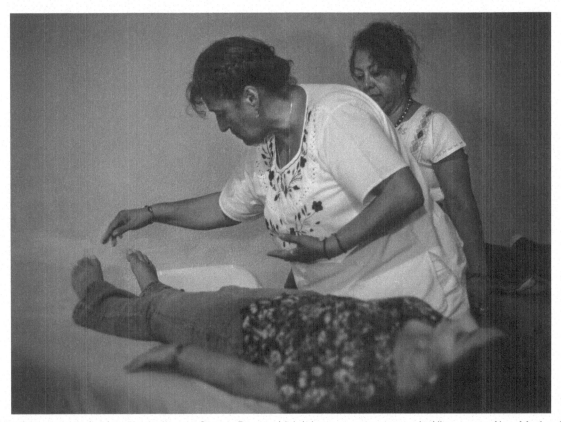

Maria del Carmen Ayala (left) and her colleague Carmen Ramírez (right) do an energy treatment in Albuquerque, New Mexico. In this image, Maria del Carmen moves her hands over the patient's body, like a human X-ray, to detect ailments. Once detected, Maria del Carmen and her friend direct the energy to that area by hovering their hands above it.

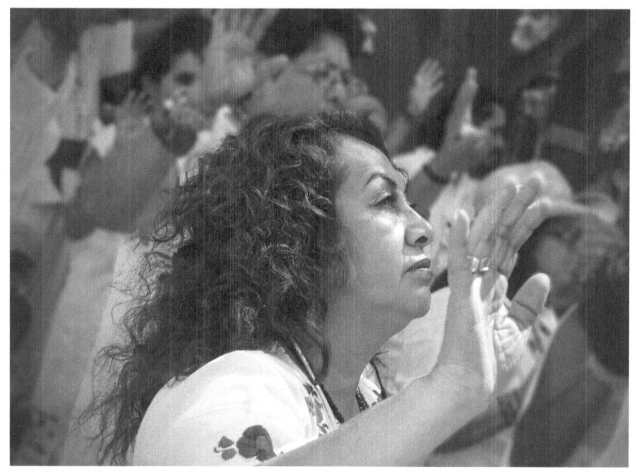

Carmen Ramírez participates in a community ceremony that honors the four cardinal directions, the Father Sky and the Mother Earth in Santa Fe, New Mexico.

MARIA LUCIA FLORES

Maria Lucia became interested in traditional medicine because, like other healers, she was ill. She was born in Mexico City and has lived there most of her life. Her introduction to traditional medicine was through energy work, *limpias,* and osteopathy. She studied at the holistic medicine school in Cuernavaca and the Mexican School of Osteopathy.

Maria's great aunt was a healer and herbalist who motivated her to become a traditional healer. Before the age of 15, she had not seen a physician, since her *curandera* relative treated her of colds, fevers, injuries, and even performed minor surgery.

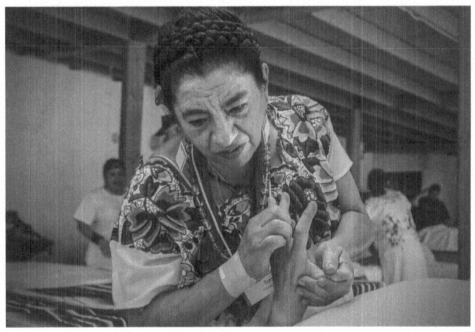

Maria Lucia Flores helps a patient at a traditional health fair in Santa Fe, New Mexico. Maria believes that we are brought to this world to help others including animals. At home, she treats her own dogs with energy work.

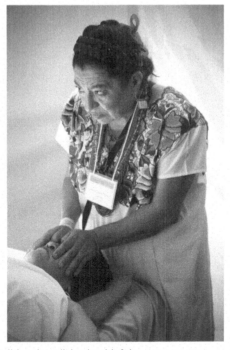

Maria Lucia Flores treats a woman at a traditional medicine health fair.

DR. YSAMUR FLORES

Dr. Ysamur Flores is a university professor at Otis College who received his PhD from the University of California in Los Angeles and researched and published on African diaspora religions in the New World. He comes from three generations of priests in the Lucumi Afro-Caribbean healing traditions. He has attended the summer curanderismo class and has recorded a video for the online program, "Global Perspectives and Influences of Curanderismo." He is an expert on the Puerto Rican Afro-Caribbean healing traditions and at the University of New Mexico demonstrated an Osain (considered the God of all healing plants) spiritual cleansing. In his recorded *limpia*, Dr. Flores uses the *Vencedor*/Lilac Chaste Tree plant leaves that emit positive vibrations and absorb negative ones. He also used a red square fabric that symbolizes life and a black fabric for death.

He does a second *limpia*/cleansing reflected in the following photo using a plate to pick up the energy from the person followed by burning a candle and analyzing the patterns of the wax.

Dr. Flores is committed in his beliefs, heritage, and culture and as a cultural anthropologist. This is reflected in his writings, research, and practices.

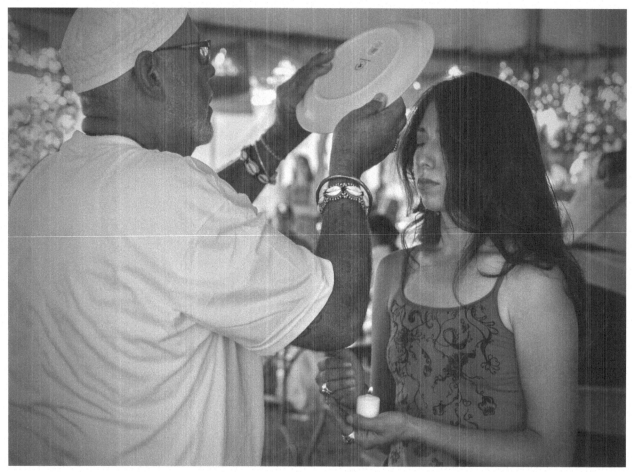

Dr. Ysamur Flores, of Puerto Rican heritage, is a professor and a traditional healer/ Lucumi Priest who is performing an Osain spiritual healing at a traditional healing fair. In this session, the plate is used to pick up negative energy from the patient. The patterns of the wax from the candle are used to diagnose the problems. Once the session is complete, the plate is broken and the candle containing the good intentions is carried home by the patient.

DR. FELINA ORTIZ

As a nurse-midwife, Dr. Felina Ortiz specializes in women's health. She educates women about their bodies, helps them unleash their inner power, and is an activist for women's rights, including reproductive justice. She works with culturally diverse families, is an advocate for the disadvantaged, believes in a holistic traditional care, and is respectful of others' spiritual and cultural beliefs.

After practicing as a certified nurse-midwife in clinical practice with marginalized communities for eight years, Dr. Ortiz joined the University of New Mexico's College of Nursing faculty in 2011. Dr. Ortiz led the development and implementation of prenatal group care facilitated by midwives and community health workers, in a faculty practice-based rural community health center. Currently, she leads a community maternal child health elective for undergraduate students as well as teaching Women's Health and Newborn care within the nurse-midwifery and family nurse practitioner programs.

Her clinical scholarship foci included awareness and improvement for maternal child health disparities within communities of color, as well as recruitment and support of students and faculty of color. She cocreated the New Mexico chapter of Midwives of Color and a national mentoring program that helps recruit, support, and empower Midwives of Color, promoting a positive impact within their own communities.

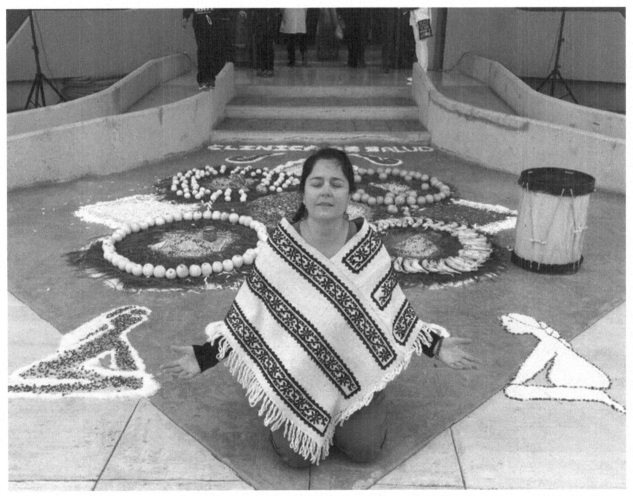

Dr. Felina Ortiz is at the Intercultural University in San Felipe del Progreso, Mexico, at a Midwifery Conference on merging traditional childbirth with allopathic practices. She is part of a delegation led by healers Rita Navarrete and Toñita Gonzales representing the Nonprofit *La Cultura Cura.* Felina Ortiz. Photo courtesy of Felina Ortiz.

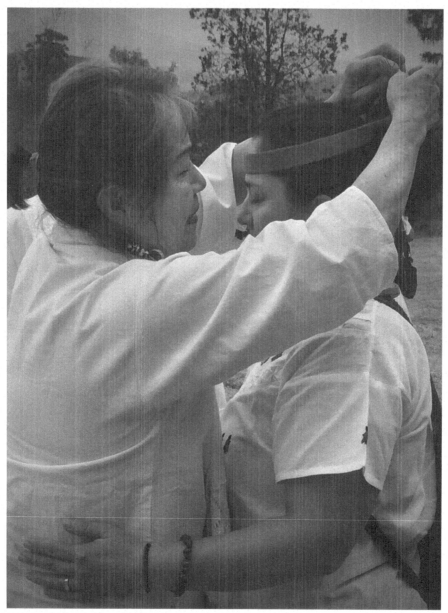

Dr. Felina Ortiz is blessed and gifted by Rita Navarrete, with a traditional red sash for the head and waist, for protection, and as a sign of being a carrier of traditional medicine, at the pyramids of Cuicuilco, Mexico, during the Spring Equinox. Photo Courtesy of Toñita Gonzales.

SELMA SROKA, MD

Dr. Sroka is a native of Minneapolis, Minnesota. She completed medical training and has integrated traditional healing therapies because of their powerful tools and strength in addressing emotional and spiritual healing.

She attended medical school at the University of Minnesota and completed a three-year specialty program in family medicine.

She was a student of the late *curandera* Elena Avila before studying with Rita Navarrete and Toñita Gonzales. Elena took Dr. Sroka and others to sacred sites in Mexico City and introduced them to traditional healer Rita Navarrete which led to her studies in Mexico City, and has continued her mission of integrating allopathic with traditional medicine.

She participates in a Latino organization called "*El Centro*" in Minneapolis where she assisted the group in initiating a nine-month tutorial called "Fundamentals of Traditional Healing." This program seeks to train the community on the tools and therapies of traditional medicine.

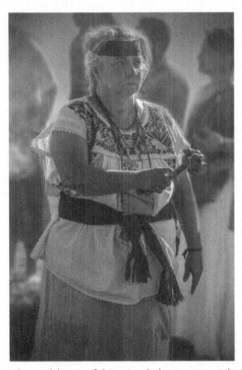

Dr. Sroka participates in a ceremony to bless the participants of the *curanderismo* course at the University of New Mexico in Albuquerque.

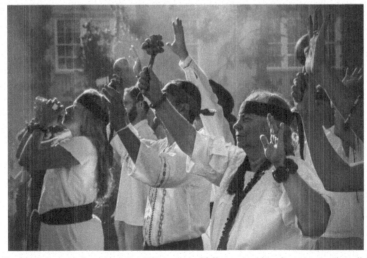

Dr. Sroka, physician at the Health Sciences Center at the University of Minnesota, has incorporated traditional and allopathic medicine. In this image, she participates in a community ceremony at the University of New Mexico.

BOB VETTER

Bob is a cultural anthropologist who has been conducting fieldwork in the area of spirituality and healing among the Southern Plains tribes since 1980. He has been adopted into families in the Cheyenne, Kiowa, and Comanche tribes. His adopted grandfather was Oliver Pahdopony, the last medicine man of the Comanches. Along with his adopted Kiowa uncle and medicine man Richard Tartsah Sr., he authored the book "Big Bow: The Spiritual Life and Teachings of a Kiowa Family." Through his organization Journeys Into American Indian Territory, he has been sharing experimental workshops with thousands of people since 1987. Bob is a healer practitioner of *curanderismo* and maintains a *temazcal* as a part of his spiritual community in New York.

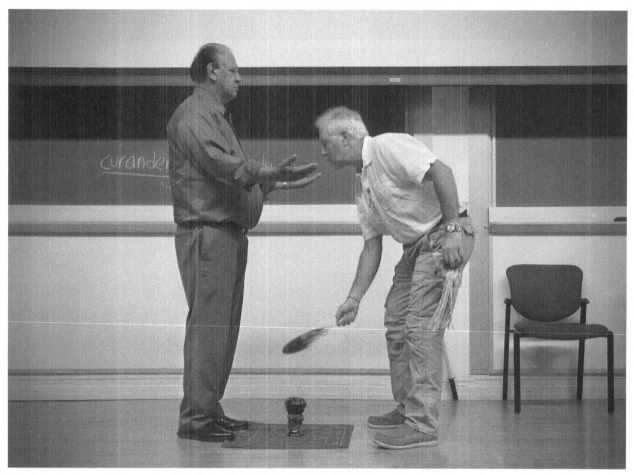

Bob demonstrates an indigenous spiritual cleansing with a sacred feather at the University of New Mexico. Dr. Eliseo "Cheo" Torres is the recipient of the cleansing. Bob prayed for the well-being of Dr. Torres and asked for healing, balance, and harmony in his life.

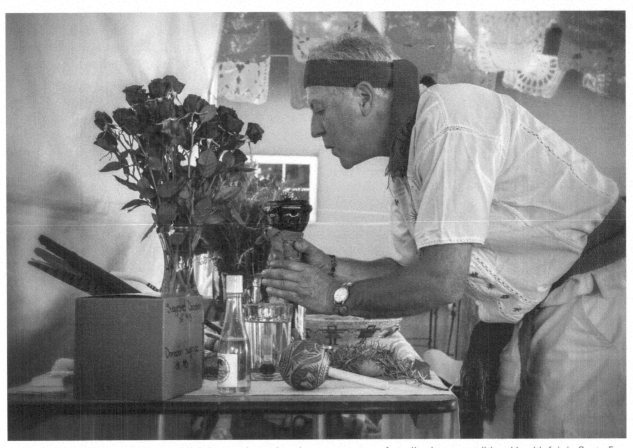

Bob is preparing his sacred space and lighting a *sahumerio* as he prepares to perform *limpias* at a traditional health fair in Santa Fe, New Mexico.

ALEX JACKSON, LMT, NCTMB

Alex is a holistic health practitioner specializing in Mayan traditional healing. For the last decade, Alex's primary focus in his practice has been on traditional ways to heal the body and spirit through the abdomen. He believes that proper balance in the core can resolve many physical ailments and emotional traumas. He sees the abdomen as the doorway in achieving balance or a "centered spirit." *Curanderismo* has been vital and has provided the missing link in health care for his patients. His objective is to bring this ancient healing wisdom to our modern world.

Alex is trained as a licensed massage therapist and is certified as a practitioner and self-care instructor in the Arvigo Techniques of Mayan Abdominal Therapy. His training also includes CranioSacral Therapy, Reiki, nutrition, prenatal massage, Chi Nei Tsang, cupping therapy, medicinal plants, and holistic counseling. Alex's journey in Mayan traditional healing has taken him to Belize, Guatemala, and Mexico, where respected *curanderos* taught him the simple but effective power of natural medicine. He trained with Dr. Rosita Arvigo of Belize, Central America, on Mayan spiritual healing and abdominal therapy and with Rita Navarrete from Mexico on the *temazcal* and *limpias*.

He is the founder and owner of Centered Spirit, LLC, a clinic specializing in abdominal health, therapeutic massage, and traditional healing, located in Kansas City, Missouri. There he treats women with menstrual and reproductive issues such as painful periods, irregular cycles, tipped uterus, infertility, and bladder pain.

He teaches workshops on abdominal health and Mayan traditional healing throughout the year and is a self-care teacher for the Arvigo Institute.

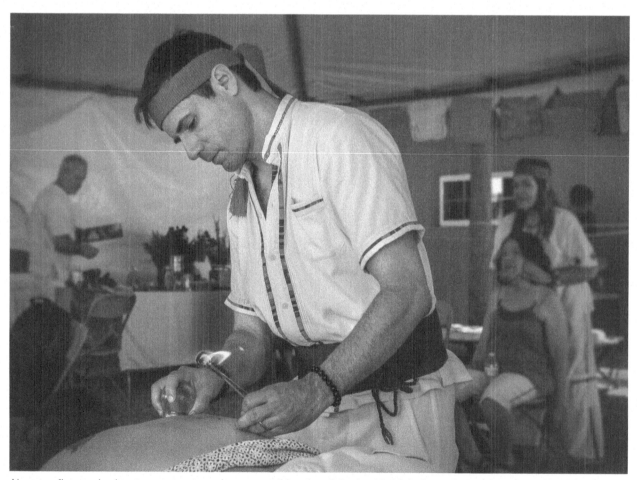

Alex uses fire cupping/*ventosas* to treat a patient at a traditional medicine health fair in Santa Fe, New Mexico.

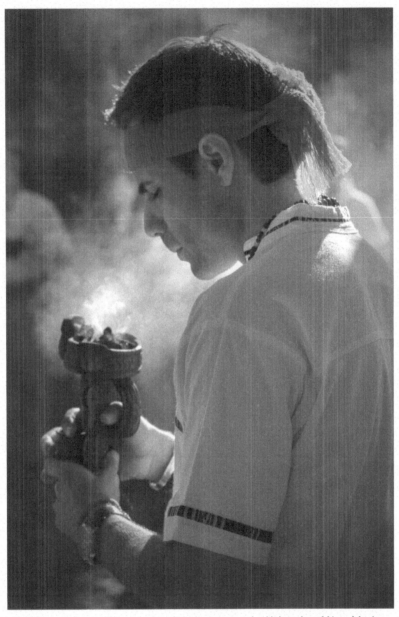

Alex prepares his *sahumerio* before taking part in a community ceremony at the University of New Mexico.

KATHERINE WHITE

Katherine was born in Minnesota and moved to Albuquerque, New Mexico, in 1997. She is a retired registered nurse and spent 27 years in practice. Toward the end of her tenure, she became disenchanted with western medicine and wanted to study herbalism. Once retired, she dedicated her life to studying medicinal herbs.

She met Maestra Laura and became an apprentice with her community group, Kalpulli Teocalli Ollin. Her introduction to *curanderismo* came in 2007, when she attended the traditional medicine summer class. It served as a link to spiritual fulfillment and also provided a new direction in her career as a health professional.

Katherine has been associated with the organization Kalpulli Teocalli Ollin since 2006 and is an herbalist and facilitator of Mexican sweat lodge sessions. In addition, she performs *limpias*, Reiki, and chakra balancing.

She is aware of the holistic nature of *curanderismo* and grows many of her own medicinal herbs. She understands that this type of medicine requires commitment and effort on the part of the person that is seeking the healing.

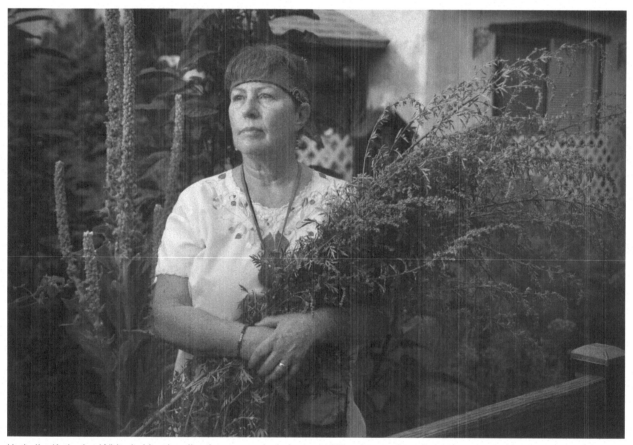

Herbalist Katherine White holds a bundle of mugwort plants harvested from her garden where she grows over 50 medicinal plants. She uses her knowledge of plants and her studies in *curanderismo* to serve the community of Albuquerque, New Mexico.

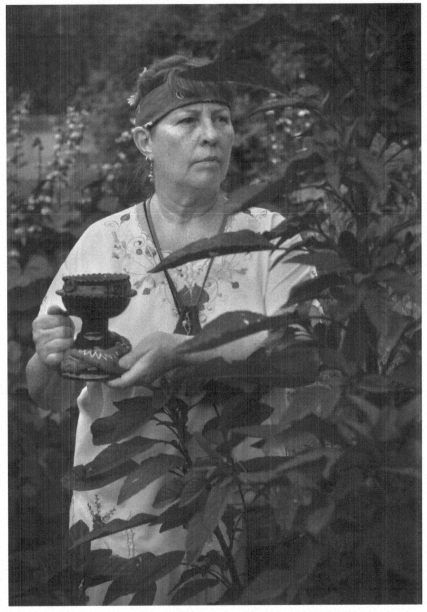

Katherine White at her home garden in Albuquerque, New Mexico. She holds her *sahumerio*, which she uses to do spiritual cleansings.

KIMBERLY "KIM" HART, NCBTMB, NGH, MINISTER

Kim has a passion for Natural Health and Indigenous Healing Methods and has been practicing holistic health since 1993 when she founded Adagio Holistic Therapies, LLC. She has integrated and formed a unique method of working with clients and students employing an indigenous philosophy and techniques taught to her by the elders of Central America as well as other western and eastern traditions.

She has traveled, lived, and studied in Central America with elders of the Mayan and Aztec cultures such as Hortense Robinson, Beatrice Waight, Elena Avila, Maria Galina, Rita Navarrete, Rosita Arvigo, Juana Shish, Lise Wolfe, Matthew Wood, Julia Graves, Liz Koch, Tieraona Low Dog, Don Mei, Martin Prechtel, Mr. Harry Guy, Toñita Gonzales, and Laurencio Nunez.

Kim is an ordained minister, certified hypnotherapist, herbalist, Mayan medicine practitioner; she is board-certified in therapeutic massage and bodywork and has developed the H.A.R.T. Method: Holistic Abdominal Relief Therapy. She lives in Minnesota and she teaches internationally.

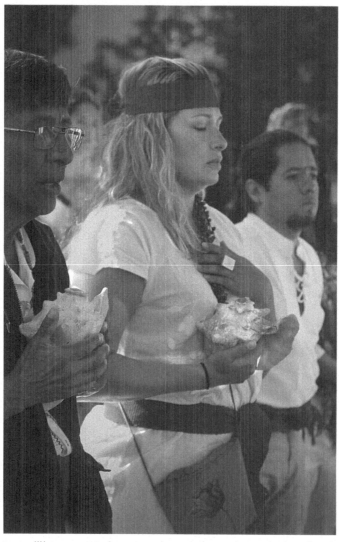

Kim is preparing to blow the *atecocolli* horn as part of a community ceremony to honor the four directions.

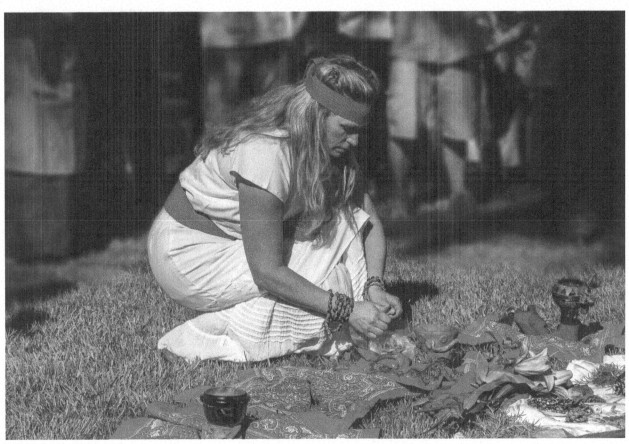

Kim is preparing *copal* incense in a sacred space with a number of *sahumerios* placed on top of traditional kerchiefs/*paliacates*.

AGUSTIN PÉREZ

Agustin is one of the few bonesetters that have survived in a traditional profession that is becoming extinct. The bonesetter was around in earlier times before osteopaths, chiropractors, and physical therapists. Like many traditional healers, Agustin, with no formal training, was an apprentice of his grandfather and father. He works with his hands, forearms, and elbows to address muscular problems and with *ventosas* for certain problems. One of the major ailments that he frequently addresses is sciatica that is associated with a painful nerve that runs from the gluteal/buttock muscles down to the feet. He addresses this problem with deep running *ventosas*. Deep means that there is a stronger pull of the skin and muscles after he sprays alcohol in a cupping glass before placing fire in the container in order to create a deeper suction on the skin.

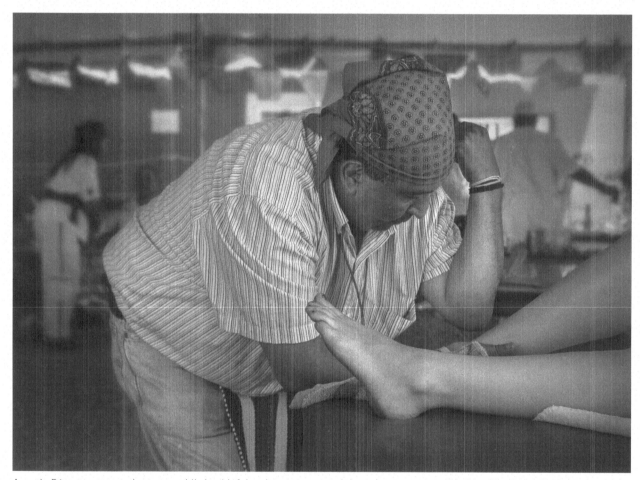

Agustin Pérez treats a patient at a public health fair using *ventosas* and deep tissue massage. He identifies himself as a bonesetter and his work consists mainly of traditional chiropractic work. Santa Fe, New Mexico.

THE REVEREND VIRGINIA MARIE RINCÓN

Virginia Marie Rincón begins her story by recognizing her ancestors. She states, "My grandmother, Maria Nestora was my first *maestra* since she would greet me with a *taquito* or a bit of *pan dulce*/sweet bread after school, and slowly coax out the stories of the emotional injuries I was forced to endure. She knew me better than anyone in the world and noticed how racism and inequality affected me. Wrapped in her gentleness and caring, she would lay me down and use a broom made out of herbs and clear away the day's trauma. Through her loving example I learned about the necessity and benefits of spiritual healing in the world."

After 20 years of nursing, she received a degree in social work from St. Edward's University in Austin, Texas, and in 1997 a Masters in Divinity from the Episcopal Divinity School in Cambridge, Massachusetts. She was ordained as an Episcopal priest in 2005. She founded *Tengo Voz*, a nonprofit organization dedicated to the empowerment and leadership of Latina women in Maine.

Currently, she has relocated to Albuquerque, New Mexico, and says of her clients that, "their healing promotes my own healing. I promote "spiritual justice" in my practice. We must do right by our spirits if we are to be whole and able to do what our calling requires."

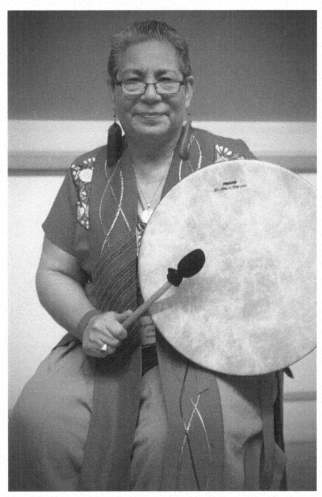

The Reverend Virginia Marie Rincón presented a healing drumming session at the University of New Mexico for the students of the *curanderismo* course. In her healing practice, she connects to the spirit of the patient and to her own to create an interconnection.

MACLOVIA SÁNCHEZ DE ZAMORA

Maclovia is an herbalist/*yerbera* who started working at Ruppe Drug store in Albuquerque in 1981. She was born in Belen, New Mexico, and has lived primarily in the central part of the state.

Her initiation in traditional medicine happened as a child in Belen. Her stepmother's mother was a midwife and *curandera* who attended to many births in Belen, Lincoln County, and other places in New Mexico.

From her stepmother, Maclovia learned about herbs of New Mexico by going to the countryside and collecting them. She remembers using some local medicinal plants like Swamp Root/*Yerba del Manso*, Osha Root/*Chuchupate*, and Spearmint/*Yerba Buena*.

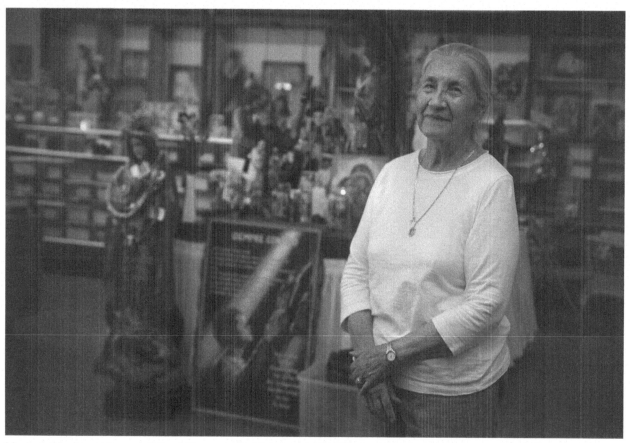

Maclovia Sánchez de Zamora at Ruppe Drug store in Albuquerque, New Mexico. She is a *yerbera* and *consejera* who has worked at Ruppe Drugs for over 30 years. Her store offers a wide selection of herbs, essential oils, and tinctures. In addition, a visitor can find amulets, statuettes, posters, and books about Mexican American traditions and saints.

CHAPTER 5

Curanderos(as) of Tomorrow

There is much interest in the field of *curanderismo*, especially by young professionals and some university students who are interested in how their ancestor's medicine can be incorporated into their profession. Through the creation of a new healing system that integrates modern and traditional medicine, they strive to empower marginalized communities to take control of their own health needs using a new and inexpensive medicine of tomorrow.

The images and narratives in this section tell the story of how these young people have devoted time and energy to study both in Mexico and in the United States with some well-known *curanderos(as)* who have dedicated their lives to the traditional medicine field. Most of these *curanderos(as)* are instructors at *Centro de Desarrollo Humano Hacia la Comunidad*/Center for Community Human Development directed by Dr. Arturo Ornelas.

Other opportunities to learn about the medicine of the ancestors include short summer classes and online semester courses that I have been offering at the University of New Mexico. All of the **"Curanderos(as) of Tomorrow"** have been students in the summer *curanderismo* course. Dr. Terry Crowe, professor in the occupational therapy program, also offers a hands-on summer course on traditional medicine in Oaxaca, Mexico. Some of the professionals featured in this section have traveled with Dr. Crowe to learn hands-on traditional therapies with Mexican *curanderos* such as Laurencio Nuñez and others. The modalities of healing being taught to these professionals from the United States include the preparation of medicinal plants in tinctures, microdosages, salves, and pomades. Many have become proficient in *sobadas*, *temazcal*, *ventosas*, *limpias*, *manteadas*, and many other therapies.

They have had instructors from the United States and Mexico such as Rita Navarrete, Toñita Gonzales, Doris Ortiz, Velia Herrera, Tana Sánchez, Tomas Enos, Juan Carlos Solana, Lety Amaro, Bob Vetter, Alex Jackson, and others. These *curanderos* of tomorrow will soon join the previously mentioned healers of nowadays in teaching and in creating a new paradigm of healing where traditional medicine will be integrated into their healing practices.

You will enjoy learning about the healers of tomorrow with the provided images and information about their activities in healing ceremonies and/or modalities. These committed individuals represent a number of professions, who incorporate traditional healing therapies into their job descriptions.

In this section, you will learn about Dr. Tom Chávez who is professor at the University of New Mexico and has incorporated his traditional medicine training into his educational and family counseling program. Dr. Chávez has trained with Toñita Gonzales. Julie McGarahan is a retired educator who was adopted as a young child, but states, "I have now reclaimed "genetic memory" of my Mexican ancestors who practice *curanderismo*." One of her goals is to construct a *temazcal*/sweat lodge next to a traditional medicine clinic in Bernalillo, New Mexico.

Rosalba de las Flores was raised in Ciudad Juarez, Chihuahua, Mexico, and now lives in Santa Fe, New Mexico. Her goal as a social worker is to use her skills in traditional medicine to treat her community with compassion in order to improve the lives of others. Raquel Catalina Reyna from Texas has a similar goal of serving her community. She is proud of her indigenous roots that are of U.S. Lipan Apache and Mexican Huasteca Potosi and has founded her own wellness company. Jeff Bazanele is from Colorado with parents from Italy and Mexico. He learned about medicinal plants from his grandparents. His degree is in Occupational Therapy from the University of New Mexico's Health Sciences Center where one of his courses on *curanderismo* was in Oaxaca, Mexico. He also studied in Cuernavaca.

Maria Cristina Renner from Indianapolis, Indiana, learned about *curanderismo* from her Mexican grandmother. She is a certified massage therapist who has taken a number of classes in Mexico and has incorporated traditional medicine therapies into her practice. Michael Guzzio, a former pastor, was born in New York. He is also well trained in Mexican traditional medicine, which he fuses with the Sicilian folk medicine of his background.

These young professionals are committed to providing services to the community and improving the lives of others. All give recognition to their Mexican ancestors and culture, and most mentioned how they learned from their grandparents. Because of the healers of tomorrow, we will enjoy a healthier and happier way of life.

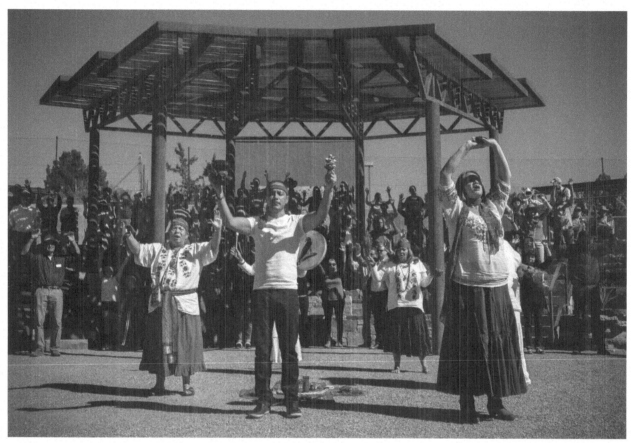

The practice of *curanderismo* is changing in the United States as this image from the Santa Fe Botanical Garden's Community Ceremony demonstrates. Left to right: Rev. Virginia Marie Rincón, Professor Dr. Tom Cháves, Job Counselor Cecilia Martínez Howard, and Social Worker Rosalba de las Flores. All have incorporated traditional healing into their professions.

TOM ANTHONY CHÁVEZ, PHD

Dr. Tom Chávez was born and raised in the Northern New Mexican town of Española, where Chicano/Hispano traditions have defined the way of life for centuries. Traditional medicine has been an important part of his cultural identity. He has witnessed practices from prescribing herbal teas for minor ailments, to the role of traditional healers in his community.

These experiences have influenced his career path in psychology and counseling, a field in which he teaches at the University of New Mexico. His goal is to integrate the traditional healing practices of the American Southwest and Mexico with western modes of counseling.

Dr. Chávez has been active in the art of traditional healing for over six years by studying and practicing alongside New Mexican and Mexican healers alike. According to Tom, his study and practice "flourished after attending the Traditional Medicine course at the University of New Mexico." He now focuses on *sobadas, ventosas,* and the facilitation of *temazcal* sessions.

He has presented to professional and community organizations on the topics of health education and well-being through a Hispano and indigenous lens. He has done so in collaboration with Remembering Ancestors, Inspiring Community, and Empowering Self (R.A.I.C.E.S.), an organization founded by Tonita Gonzales mentioned in a previous chapter.

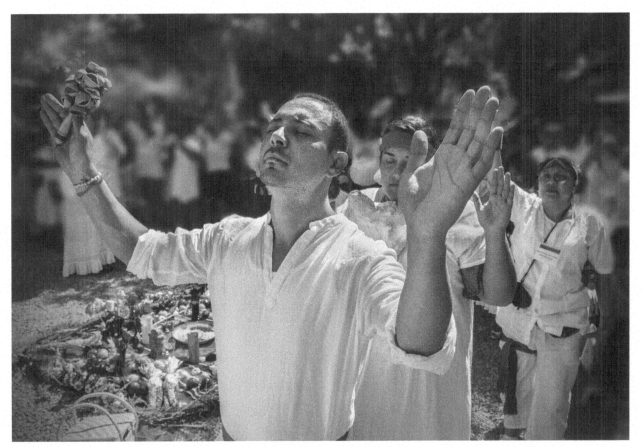

Dr. Chávez uses a traditional incense burner to bless the participants of the traditional medicine course at the University of New Mexico. His involvement in traditional medicine has led him to embrace a mission to help the community of New Mexico and beyond find holistic healing.

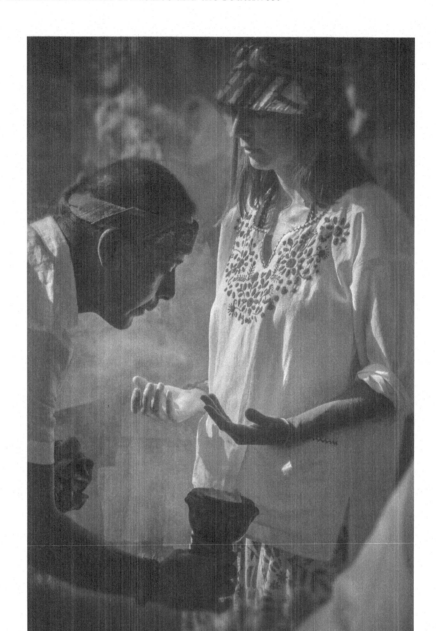

Dr. Chávez participates in a ceremony to honor the four cardinal directions. On the ground, there is a sacred space containing symbolic objects such as corn, flowers, prehispanic statuettes, herbs, plants, candles, and baskets. Santa Fe, New Mexico.

JULIE MCGAHARAN

After a teaching career, Julie decided to study and become a traditional healer. She attended seminars at the Center for Community Human Development in Cuernavaca. She followed up with a second training experience with a course on traditional medicine offered by Dr. Terry Crowe with the Occupational Therapy Department of the Health Sciences Center at the University of New Mexico. During this course, she met the well-known *curandero* of Oaxaca, Laurencio Nuñez, who became her mentor. Julie now grows her medicinal plants, works with balancing the chakras, and does crystal work, *sobadas*, *platicas*, and yoga therapy.

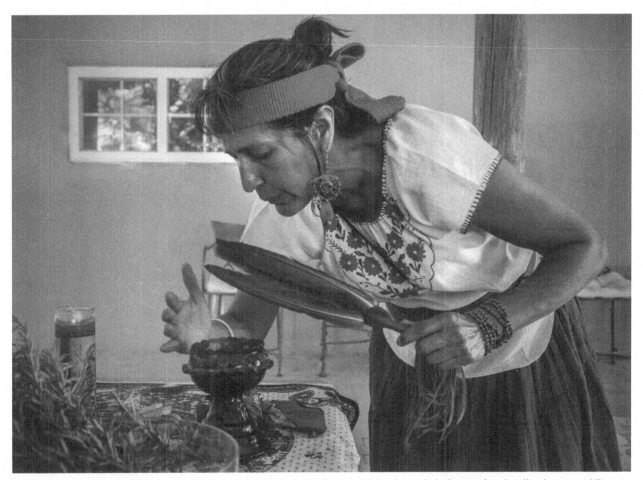

Julie prepares her healing instruments such as candles, feathers, *Romero*, and *sahumerio,* before performing *limpias* at a public health fair. Santa Fe, New Mexico.

ROSALBA DE LAS FLORES

Rosalba grew up in the border city of Ciudad Juarez, Chihuahua, Mexico, in an environment where family was an integral part of life. She describes the proximity of family as being like "water to the earth; without it, life is a struggle." Her maternal grandmother, Doña Angela Roman, practiced traditional medicine on the family during times of sickness and need. Rosalba considers her mother and grandmother role models who taught her the values of compassion, healing, perseverance, and strength.

She considers herself a dreamer, idealistic, and a humanitarian traditional healer who understands that society can focus too much on materialistic pursuits, mundane routines and self-preservation. Yearning to make this world a better place, she learned to explore the mysteries of the human experience and connect with the spiritual world. In addition, Rosalba draws inspiration in her healing work from looking closely into nature. She encourages us to look into the wonders of nature to find beauty and healing.

Rosalba is a social worker, mother, friend, artist, and a traditional healer. Her perception and intuition lead her to treat people with compassion and to encourage positive transformation.

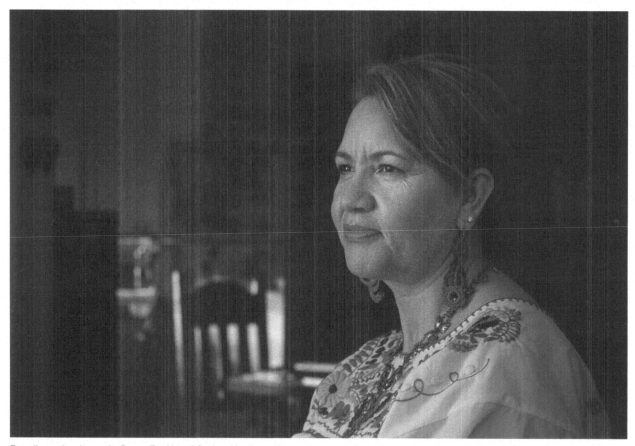

Rosalba at her home in Santa Fe, New Mexico. Her home is a sanctuary where she finds peace and inspiration. She carefully selects and displays objects such as family photographs, pre-Columbian statuettes, and drums that serve as symbolic objects for healing.

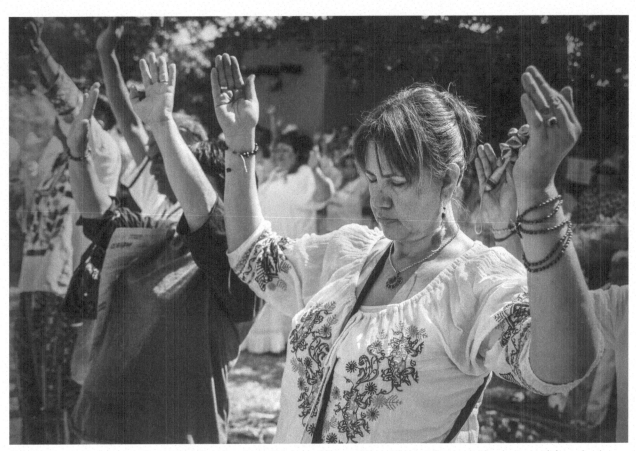

Rosalba is aware of the role that spirituality plays in traditional medicine. When doing healing work, she does not claim to heal people. Instead, she asks for guidance and assistance from the spirit of God. Her role is that of a conduit between the healing energy of God and the patient, which can sometimes involve trance.

RAQUEL CATALINA REYNA

Raquel traces her ancestors to the Lipan Apache indigenous tribe of Texas and to the Huasteca Potosi Indian community of the state of San Luis Potosi, Mexico. As a youngster, she found herself helping people heal themselves. She was first called a *curandera*/healer at the age of 17 by her uncle Gregory Gomez.

At first, she was offended by the name *curandera* since she thought involved witchcraft. However, she eventually learned that the term refers to a person with good intentions to help others heal.

Raquel holds a Bachelor of Science in Nutrition, Human Development and Family Studies and American Sign Language from Texas Tech University in Lubbock, Texas. In addition, she studied at the first ever pilot master's program of Maharishi Ayurveda and Integrative Medicine at Maharishi University of Management.

She founded a wellness company, in which she acts as an integrative health specialist and registered yoga teacher. Raquel has worked with troubled teens and people who have suffered from post-traumatic stress disorder and substance abuse. Her goal is to use her talents to help people heal themselves on Indian reservations and in the state of San Luis Potosi in Mexico.

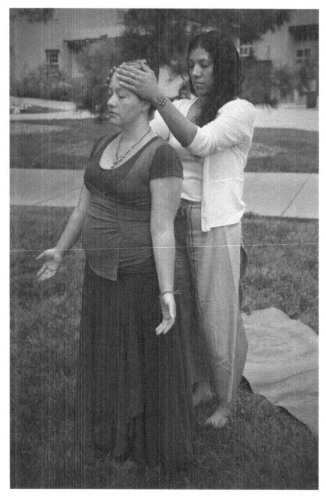

Raquel Catalina Reyna (right) applying lessons learned from the Traditional Medicine class at the University of New Mexico.

JEFF R. BAZANELE

Jeff was born to an Italian father and a Mexican mother in Pueblo, Colorado, and was raised in the "four corners" area of the Southwest. His journey in *curanderismo* began through his maternal grandparents who lived in the four corners (a region in the Southwest where Arizona, New Mexico, Colorado, and Utah meet). As a child, they taught Jeff to identify, harvest, and prepare herbs, roots, fruits, vegetables, and animal meats for medicinal uses from the local environment. Jeff referred to this knowledge as *"la sabiduría del pueblo,"* or "the wisdom of the common folk," without knowing that many people call it *"curanderismo."* In his college years, Jeff was introduced to traditional medicine or *curanderismo*.

Upon graduation, he decided to fully embrace his background and roots by studying in Cuernavaca, Mexico. When he returned to the United States, he moved to Albuquerque where he found the proper environment to practice *sobadas* and other forms of traditional medicine for the community. Once in Albuquerque, he partnered with Toñita Gonzales to help start the traditional medicine organization R.A.I.C.E.S. According to Jeff, R.A.I.C.E.S. "reflects the principles of *curanderismo* by empowering others to regain and better their own well-being/*bienestar*." In his practice, Jeff hopes to integrate occupational therapy with *curanderismo* to create a model of health care dedicated to well-being.

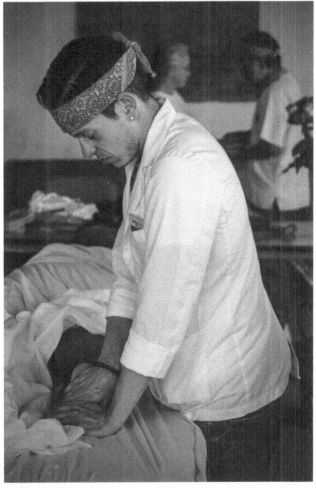

Jeff provides energetic massage at a public health fair in Santa Fe, New Mexico.

MARIA CRISTINA RENNER, MS, MPA, CMT

Maria's first introduction to *curanderismo* was through her Mexican grandmother who grew a medicinal herb garden. As an infant, Maria learned to appreciate vibrant flowers as her initiation in the world of traditional medicine. Her grandmother used traditional healing techniques such as *limpia de huevos*/cleansings with eggs on her family and with her neighbors. She has fond memories of her grandmother speaking with the plants and wildlife.

Throughout her life, Maria experienced profound healing, transformation, connection, and beauty though *curanderismo*, both as a client and as a practitioner. *Curanderismo* helped her through moments of deep trauma as a way of nourishing her soul, leading to greater wisdom and empowerment. Because of these experiences, Maria has been fascinated with the tremendous healing capability of indigenous medicine and has participated in numerous advanced trainings, apprenticeships, and mentorships with teachers and elders both across the United States and internationally.

She currently lives in Indianapolis, Indiana, where she is an herbalist, massage therapist, Mayan medicine practitioner, and Mayan abdominal massage therapist. She practices various fire cupping techniques, flower essence therapies, and spiritual cleansings. She dedicates her practice to the spirit of her grandparents and indigenous ancestors.

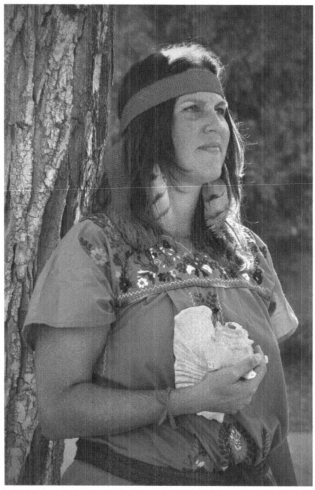

Maria Cristina Renner directs Abalone Holistic Therapies in Indianapolis, Indiana, where she incorporates *curanderismo* traditions into her practice. The clinic provides services including fire cupping pregnancy and postpartum therapies, Mayan abdominal therapy and others.

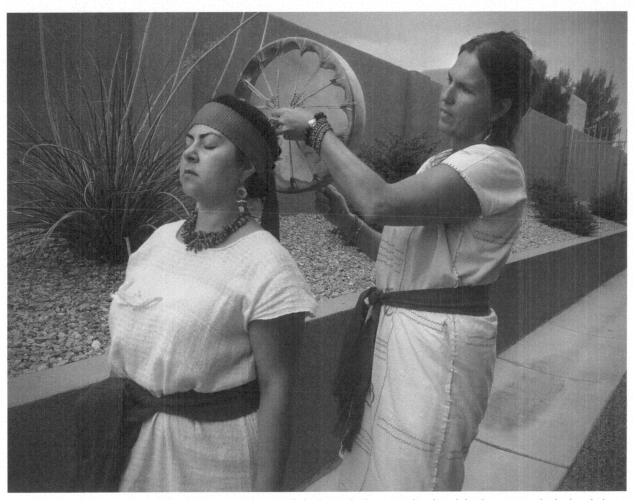

Maria Cristina Renner performs a limpia using sound, aromatic herbs, and other natural tools to bring harmony to the body, mind, and spirit.

MICHAEL GUZZIO

Michael is part Sicilian and was born in Buffalo, New York. As a former pastor, Michael traveled internationally to places such as Mexico and the United Kingdom. His journey in *curanderismo* began when a *curandera* asked him to train with her. After training for eight years, he was given permission to do his own work. In his practice, which is comprised mostly of *limpias* and *temazcal* sessions, he finds inspiration, as he does in his ministry and his Sicilian heritage.

According to Michael, Sicilian spiritual cleanses are similar to *limpias* in the Mexican-American tradition. Many times, holy water, rosemary, basil, mint, sage, crucifixes, and eggs are used in both styles of *limpias*. The egg is also used in Sicilian *limpias* to diagnose the type of spiritual ailment the patient has. Similarly, rituals and prayers are used to cleanse people from negative energy.

In his *limpias*, he uses selenite crystal, which he calls "a master crystal." According to Michael, selenite crystals are strong and good for clearing energy, and they help connect people with their high self, their spiritual guides, and their angels.

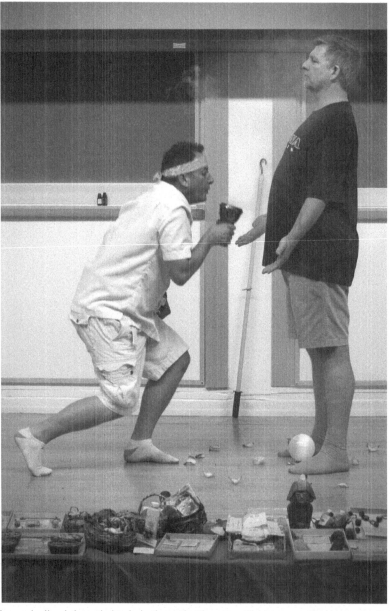

Michael performs a Sicilian-style *limpia* intended to help the patient's energy field or aura. This cleansing helps connect with divine love and cut cords from the past. In his *limpias*, Michael acts as a conduit between divine love and the patient.

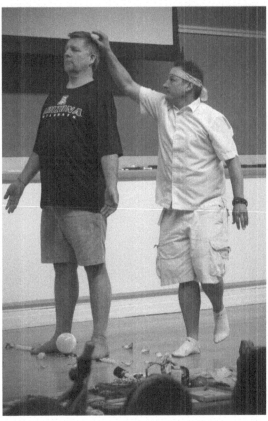

According to Michael, in the Sicilian belief system, Archangel Michael is involved in many ceremonies and rituals. In his work, he intends to channel the spirit of Archangel Michael, Christ consciousness, and other angelic energies.

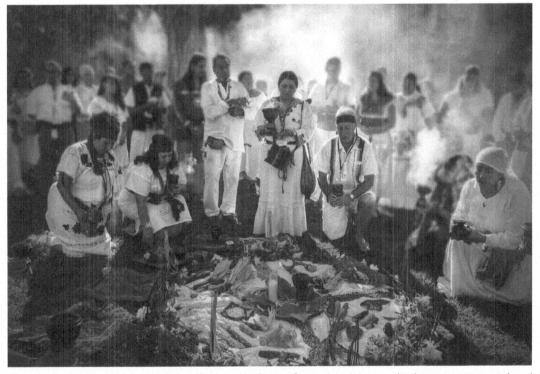

This image is part of a ceremony honoring Mother Earth with a Sacred Space that shows a union between two countries, the United States and Mexico in preservation of *curanderismo* traditional medicine. If merged with modern, allopathic medicine, this could be the medicine of tomorrow.

Conclusion

Imanol and I hope that this publication has given you an appreciation of a healing tradition that has survived for hundreds of years. It has now evolved and changed, both in Mexico and in the United States, in order to meet the needs of the new generation. The history of traditional medicine is presented by Imanol's excellent photographs that have captured ritual, healing, therapy, and ceremony done by a diverse group of healers from two countries and one with Puerto Rican heritage.

We have offered you an overview of *curanderismo* which includes the definition of Mexican traditional medicine and the history of *curanderismo,* beginning with the arrival of the Spaniards to the New World. In this section, we have given you the types of *curanderos(as)* and the three levels of healing: the material, spiritual, and mental. There are a number of examples for each of the three levels in order to clarify their meaning.

We have divided the publication into four sections or chapters beginning with *curanderos(as)* of yesteryear, of recent times, of nowadays, and of tomorrow. These four sections offer photographs of a diversity of healers by country, region, gender, and age. The *curanderos(as)* from Mexico have been the change agents of the American healers of nowadays, and these charismatic individuals have influenced the healers of tomorrow.

In the first section, we have presented **Curanderos(as) of Yesteryear: The Three Great Ones** who were active in the late 1800s and early 1900s. They were Don Pedrito Jaramillo, Niño Fidencio, and Teresita. All three Mexican healers have had an influence in the United States. Both Don Pedrito and Teresita came to this country and continued their healing practices here. They influenced hundreds of Americans while the healings of El Niño Fidencio continue being practiced by thousands of followers called Fidencistas throughout Mexico and the United States. We discovered that all three *curanderos(as)* did not know each other, but all had commonalities such as being charismatic, noble, sincere, and being considered folk saints (not church recognized and canonized) while they were alive.

In the second section, **Curanderos(as) of Recent Times: Impacting the United Mexico,** we have learned about four *curanderos(as)* who are no longer with us but left a legacy. Two of them, Elena Avila and Alberto Salinas, Jr., have authored books on their life while publications on Jewel Babb discuss her contributions and commitments to healing those in need. Felipa Sanchez was a gentle but powerful healer with a psychic gift. All four of these healers died within the last few years and had an impact in Mexico as well as in the United States. Jewel Babb and Alberto Salinas, Jr. lived on the United States/Mexican border and saw patients from both countries while Felipe had a clinic in Mexico and New Mexico. Elena, born in El Paso, United States/Mexican border, trained and collaborated with a number of *curanderos(as)* from Mexico.

In the third section, **Curanderos(as) of Nowadays: Creating a New Tradition Healing Model**, we have enjoyed a number of photographs of healers from Mexico and the United States who come from a number of states in both countries. The difference between both countries is that the Mexican *curanderos(as)* are committed to their profession full time and most of them direct traditional health clinics while the American healers have a number of other professions such as a retired nurse, university professor, social worker, religious leader, massage therapist, and a physician. They have incorporated traditional healing therapies into their professions. Most of the American healers have learned traditional use of plants and rituals from the Mexican *curanderos(as),* and they live in states such as New York, Missouri, Minnesota, Texas, and New Mexico. All of the healers from both countries are creating a new healing model of combining modern medicine with the traditional one in order to meet the needs of their communities, especially the immigrants who come from Mexico and other Latin American countries.

The final section, **Curanderos(as) of Tomorrow**, includes a number of young professionals who have trained with *curanderos(as)* of nowadays and have also incorporated the traditional therapies into their professions. Most of these committed individuals recognize their grandparents who first introduced them to traditional medicine through the usage of medicinal plants or rituals. They have been successful in incorporating many healing modalities into their professions, which include being a university professor, occupational therapist, social worker, retired educator, and a health specialist. Just as the healers of nowadays, these committed professionals are already creating a new health model that will improve the lives of others.

All of the healers mentioned in these publications are committed to helping others and to doing community health services. They have realized that they will help as much as possible and will use the judgment to refer patients to allopathic practitioners when the need arises. However, a simple plant or a *limpia* may be what is needed to address serious health problems.

References

Avila, E. (1999). *Woman Who Glows in the Dark*. New York: Putnam.

Babb, J. & Littledog, P. (2010). *Border Healing Woman: The Story of Jewel Babb as Told to Pat Littledog*. Austin: University of Texas Press.

Gates, W. (2012). *An Aztec Herbal: The Classic Codex of 1552*. North Chelmsford: Courier Corporation.

Salinas, A. (2011). *The Border Healer: My Life as a Curandero*. Bloomington: Author House.

Torres, E. (2005). *Curandero: A Life in Mexican Folk Healing*. Albuquerque: University of New Mexico Press.

Torres, E. (2006). *Healing with Herbs and Rituals: A Mexican Tradition*. Albuquerque: University of New Mexico Press.

Zavaleta, A. & Salinas, A. (2009). *Curandero Conversations: El Niño Fidencio, Shamanism and Healing Traditions of the Borderlands*. Bloomington: Author House.